Evaluating health services' effectiveness

Evaluating health services' effectiveness

A guide for health professionals, service managers and policy makers

A. S. St Leger
H. Schnieden
J. P. Walsworth-Bell

Open University Press
Milton Keynes • Philadelphia

To the memory of the late Professor Archie Cochrane

Open University Press
Celtic Court
22 Ballmoor
Buckingham
MK18 1XW

and

1900 Frost Road, Suite 101
Bristol, PA 19007, USA

First published 1992

British Library Cataloguing-in-Publication Data

Evaluating health services' effectiveness:
A guide for health professionals, service managers
and policy makers.
  I. St Leger, A. S.   II. Schnieden, H.
  III. Walsworth-Bell, J. P.

  ISBN 0-335-09357-4
  ISBN 0-335-09356-6 pbk

Library of Congress Cataloging-in-Publication Data

Evaluating health services' effectiveness: a guide for health professionals,
service managers, and policy makers/ A.S.
St. Leger, H. Schnieden, J.P. Walsworth-Bell.
  p.   cm.
Includes bibliographical references and index.
  ISBN 0-335-09356-6 (pbk.)   ISBN 0-335-09357-4 (hbk.)
  1. Medical care—Evaluation. 2. Public health—Evaluation.
  I. St. Leger, A.S. (Anthony Selwyn), 1948- . II. Schnieden, H.
  (Harold) III. Walsworth-Bell, J.P. (Joanna Pierce), 1947-
  [DNLM: 1. Evaluation Studies. 2. Health Services—organization &
  administration.   W 84 E92]
RA399.A1E8   1991
362.1′ 0297—dc20
DNLM/DLC
for Library of Congress 91–24044 CIP

Typeset by Burns and Smith Ltd, Derby
Printed in Great Britain by St Edmundsbury Press, Bury St Edmunds

Contents

Foreword

This book is addressed to those who seek to use health service resources effectively and efficiently. Thus our intended readership includes clinicians, nurses and other health care professionals. However, these people alone do not shape health services. Therefore, our message is directed also at health service managers and other decision makers; for it is these individuals who must commission evaluation and act on its consequences.

The evaluation of the effectiveness of health services is rewarding but it is not easy. Moreover, it is not for those who seek to plough a narrow furrow with head bent and oblivious to what goes on elsewhere. It calls upon many traditional research skills. However, it differs from most areas of applied research because it cannot take place in isolation from the micropolitics and decision-making procedures of health services. It is directed to one end: informing the decision-making process. This requirement imposes a discipline upon evaluative exercises; certain kinds of information (e.g. about efficacy, effectiveness, cost, cost-effectiveness, and acceptability to the public) must be forthcoming in a systematic manner if managers and others are to make sensible choices among service options. Hitherto, much which purports to be evaluation is narrow in its intent and thus uninformative. A major purpose of this book is to show how evaluation can be broadened and used. Moreover, we shall argue that the recent reforms of the British National Health Service (NHS) not only facilitate development of the evaluative perspective but also make it imperative.

The breadth of outlook and knowledge required for the worthwhile evaluation of the effectiveness of health services poses problems. Few, if any, can be self-sufficient in all the skills required. Evaluation demands a multidisciplinary approach, e.g. from basic biological sciences, clinical science, clinical practitioners, managers, health economists, statisticians and information officers. Interdisciplinary collaboration is hard. It demands humility from the participants: they must accept that their individual disciplines do not necessarily dominate or own evaluative work. It requires a shared perspective on the role of evaluation and of its place in decision making. The participants must have an understanding of the rudiments of their colleagues' disciplines and an appreciation of their contribution to the overall task.

The outlook offered in this book was developed from our involvement in decision making in the health services and from our teaching and research in an academic setting. We are aware that those seeking to embark upon evaluation or to use the results of evaluation are often bewildered by its apparent complexity. The complexity is real but it is manageable if the task of evaluation is approached in a structured manner. The first chapter is devoted to providing a working definition of the evaluation of the effectiveness of health services and to placing evaluation in context. The second chapter provides a general structure for thinking about evaluation; it elaborates the very important concepts of goals, aims and objectives, it defines levels of evaluation, and it introduces some indices of outcome from evaluation. The third chapter outlines the steps involved in conducting an evaluation. It is deliberately prescriptive because we believe that those tackling evaluation for the first time require certainties rather than confusing choices. We suggest that the first three chapters be read in sequence. The remainder of the book, apart from the last chapter, consists of information about particular kinds of techniques of evaluation and of general resources. For instance, Chapter 6 includes material on testimony and case studies and Chapter 7 explores intervention studies including the randomized controlled trial.

Chapters 4, 5 and 11 are different in character. Each of these is an information resource. Chapter 4 is a comprehensive and up-to-date review of routinely available sources of information which can aid evaluation. Chapter 5 introduces basic concepts from economics. Chapter 11 presents a miscellany of methodological issues; it is based on our teaching of an introductory research methods course given at the University of Manchester. It presents material rarely found together in a single text. Moreover, it serves as an introduction to a number of statistical concepts. In so doing, it seeks not to confuse readers by forcing them to grapple with symbols at the same time as learning concepts; it is a prose account which should serve as an introduction to more detailed texts. Chapter 11 is not intended to be read straight through in one sitting. Rather, it picks up on matters raised in passing elsewhere in the book.

Chapter 12 is perhaps the most important chapter in the book. It is addressed to all readers but requires particular attention from policy makers and managers. The chapter attempts a fairly provocative analysis of faults in decision-making procedures in the prereformation NHS and shows why and how evaluation must become a central issue in future.

All the chapters should be regarded as opening doors to an extensive, fragmented and often difficult literature on aspects of evaluation. The references at the end of the chapters pick up on detail or contain examples. They have been kept as few in number as practicable. Other doors to be opened are found among the works in the further reading list at the end of the book.

Most of the examples in the book and much of the discussion in Chapter 12 relate to the NHS. This is because the NHS is the source of our daily experience and it is in this context that we can most credibly write about evaluation. Nevertheless, most of what we have to say applies to any kind of health service, nationalized or private. Thus, we hope the book will be helpful to readers elsewhere, but they will have to translate our exhortations that evaluation must be central to decision making into their own circumstances.

As indicated above, we aim to do little more than help our readers see the wood for the trees and then send them off to explore the forest. The book does not constitute a formal course in evaluation but selected reading from it could complement many existing taught courses on health service management, epidemiology, research methods and indeed evaluation. Moreover, the content should be of interest to health care professionals and managers preparing for professional examinations. To the lone and unassisted reader, we suggest that as soon as you get the gist of the disciplines upon which you will have to draw for evaluation, you should seek to bring collaborators around you.

Preface

This book is written by practising public health physicians for the many health service personnel, managers and policy makers who realize that they can no longer contemplate funding, purchasing or providing services without the insight which good evaluation gives. It has become apparent that some senior staff are uncertain how to evaluate, let alone how to interpret, the findings of many studies. Hence there is a need for guidance.

Much of our professional time is given to evaluation both in its practical application at the regional and district health authority levels and through instruction of professionals from diverse backgrounds. We draw on this experience in producing this book. Our work should be viewed as a guide book and map for unfamiliar territory. We seek to set the traveller on a secure path that avoids many of the dangers lurking in wait of the unwary. Our principal aims are to place evaluation in context and to show the traveller broader horizons which may be approached via the more technical works of others.

As we shall try to show, evaluation is necessarily a multidisciplinary task. We are not self-sufficient and we owe a great debt to many friends and colleagues who have collaborated with us in our work over the years. Many of the insights which we have tried to assemble and share in this book are owed to others and where possible we have acknowledged those debts. At this point, however, we wish to make specific acknowledgement of the following from the North Western Regional Health Authority: Mrs Chris Beswick, Typing Services Supervisor; Mrs Glenys Joyce, Secretary; Dr A. Haycox, Health Economist; Mrs S. Padden, Librarian, and to Mrs Marie Whitley, Secretary (retired) in the Department of Public Health and Epidemiology at the University of Manchester.

Chapter 1

An overview of evaluation

Introduction

This chapter is a small-scale map of territory which will be unfamiliar to some. It will indicate some of the major features of health service evaluation and show how they interrelate. We defer detailed topography and precise definition of many concepts to later chapters.

Defining evaluation

An issue we will stress time and again is the need for clarity of thought at all stages in evaluation. Not least, clarity is required in the definition of the evaluative process itself and in distinguishing evaluation from routine clinical and managerial activities. There are several ways in which a framework for thinking about evaluation may be constructed. These are analogous to slicing a cake along different dimensions or viewing a building from various angles. It matters not which particular framework is used. However, if evaluative exercises are to be successful and truly to inform clinical and managerial decision making, it is vital that some framework be agreed by both the doers and recipients of evaluation. The framework to which we adhere is as follows.

The term 'evaluate' has in general usage been defined[1] as 'ascertain the amount of; find numerical expression for'. In the context of a health service, we extend this notion to define evaluation as:

> The critical assessment, on as objective basis as possible, of the degree to which entire services or their component parts (e.g. diagnostic tests, treatments, caring procedures) fulfil stated goals.

Two elements of this definition deserve close attention. The reference to goals makes explicit a demand that evaluation requires comparison of the achievement of a service or procedure with some *standard*. This standard may be absolute or comparative. An example of the former (an absolute target) would be evaluation of a service against its stated aims, e.g. is the vaccination and immunization service achieving 90% uptake of courses of measles, mumps and rubella immunization? The latter (a comparative target) is exemplified by a clinical trial to ascertain whether a proposed innovation in treatment would be an improvement on existing treatments (e.g. greater benefits to patients, less unpleasant, cheaper). The choice of an appropriate standard can be difficult and it has a strong influence on the methods best suited to particular kinds of evaluation. A lack of standards too often leaves would-be evaluators and those who must make decisions as a result of evaluations in a morass of 'data' from which no amount of statistical sophistication can extract unequivocal answers. Sadly, the present tendency by some to seek 'quick and dirty' answers to inherently difficult questions perpetuates this and many other solecisms in the grammar of evaluation.

The second key element of our definition is *objectivity*. The more the findings of an evaluative exercise are seen to be independent of the judgements and prejudices of the evaluators and those who commissioned them, the greater the power of the exercise to influence other people. This relates closely to the demand of most sciences that experimental findings be capable of replication by different people at different times and places. However, total objectivity is not only philosophically questionable but also is impracticable. Judgement always plays a part in evaluation: in determing the terms of reference of an evaluation; in many measurement procedures; and in interpreting the findings. Thus our counsel of perfection is that necessary judgements should be made explicit and thereby subject to criticism.

In the context of this book, the interest is primarily in the evaluation of health service effectiveness. This must be reflected in the goals chosen in evaluative exercises. The evaluation of service effectiveness requires that the goals whose attainment is under examination be concerned directly, or through some known pattern of causation, to the health status or well-being of individual clients, patients or communities. In examining this further, it will be useful in the next section to review the distinction between 'structure', 'process' and 'outcome' that was developed in the writings of Donabedian.[2]

Structure, process and outcome

The context for the work of a service is largely set by its *structure*. Broadly speaking, the structure of a service is represented by its fixed costs (see Chapter 5). It comprises the relatively stable characteristics of the services: the distribution and qualifications of the personnel, and the number, size, equipment and geographic distribution of hospitals and other facilities. It also includes the way that personnel are organized, and some important components of their relationships, such as hierarchical lines of command and the integration of quality review into the day-to-day work. Taken together, these elements of the structure constitute the environment of care.

The *process* aspect of health services is how things are organized and done.

It also encompasses the manner in which activities interact. It is not too difficult to describe the structure and daily working of, say, a hospital general surgical service. Process can be examined in detail or it can be summarized in terms of indices such as hospital throughput, length of stay, turnover interval, etc. The gross effects of process may be quantified in terms of the total numbers of people from defined communities dealt with by the service in a year. The unmet demand on the service can be quantified by the size of the waiting list, though this can be a poor indicator. The service's capacity and/or efficiency in handling the demand is reflected by the distribution of waiting times of people on the waiting list. These are some examples of process.

Process has been the traditional concern of hospital administration and of most of the routine information systems devised to aid administrators. However, it is important to remember that Donabedian included aspects other than mechanistic activities in his definition of process. For him, the process of providing care included its accessibility, i.e. its relative use by different population groups; the performance of the health care provider in terms of the adequacy of the services provided, such as the appropriateness of various tests and investigations ('the diagnostic work-up'); and, finally, the set of activities that go on within and between practitioners and patients including interpersonal relationships, i.e. the behaviour of the health care staff towards the individual.

Process is very important and has, as we shall see, a bearing on the effectiveness of services. Donabedian suggests that this is because the quality of process can only be defined in normative terms; in other words, what is generally agreed to be an acceptable way of providing medical care. Also, because process involves the interaction of the component parts of the health care system it can be very difficult to measure. However, considered in isolation, matters of process are not very informative about service effectiveness.

Outcome is concerned with the impact of health services on individuals and communities. Put crudely, some benefit is expected to have accrued to a patient discharged from hospital or to a healthy individual who has undergone a course of immunization. The benefit received from contact with a service can be analysed into the benefits received from each of the component procedures of the service. Thus one may examine separately the effects of diagnostic procedures, treatments and caring services. For example, did the diagnostic tests employed materially alter the diagnostician's judgements? Was the discomfort, inconvenience and cost of the tests outweighed by the benefit to the patient (and indirectly) to the community? Could the treatments prescribed be shown to have benefited the patient and justified their cost? The overall outcome of these various procedures aggregated over all patients is a measure of the effectiveness of the service to the community.

Accreditation and quality assurance

Accreditation is a formalized procedure by which an organization, discipline or individual is deemed to have met an agreed standard. Accreditation is not a new phenomenon. For instance, the right of doctors to practise has, since the last century, been based on General Medical Council registration, which itself has been based for a considerable time on their ability to pass certain examinations at a certain standard. Conversely, medical schools following inspection have accredited certain hospitals for pre-registration training and the Royal Colleges have also accreditation standards for postgraduate training of junior medical staff. In 1919 in the USA, the College of Surgeons instituted a programme of minimum standards for all hospitals to follow. This initiative gradually evolved into the accreditation process employed by the Joint Commission on Accreditation of Hospitals which was founded in 1951.

In the future, more formal accreditation of hospitals and services is likely to occur in this country following the patterns in the USA, Canada and Australia. Broadly speaking, accredited hospitals will have to show that their governing body and general management have clearly stated goals and objectives, that there is a mission statement which defines the care values of the organization and its philosophy, that management by objective occurs for services under its care and that there are clear policies on important issues. Also, within the organization, formal procedures for implementing quality assurance will need to be seen to exist.

The quality assurance process is a clinical and managerial framework that commits staff to producing a systematic continuous process of evaluating agreed levels of care and service provision. The objectives of a quality assurance programme, as stated by a WHO working group,[3] are:

> to assure that each patient receives such a mix of diagnostic and therapeutic health services as is most likely to produce the optimum achievable health care outcome for that patient, consistent with the state of the art of medical science, and with biological factors such as the patient's age, illness, concomitant secondary diagnoses, compliance with the treatment regimen, and other related factors; with the minimal expenditure of resources necessary to accomplish this result; at the lowest achievable risk of additional injury or disability as a consequence of the treatment; and with maximal patient satisfaction with the process of care, his/her interaction with the health care system, and the results obtained.

This Group further stated that under the umbrella term 'quality assurance' there are four particular components which need to be considered:

- patient satisfaction with services provided;
- professional performance (technical quality)
- resource use (efficiency); and
- risk management (the risk of illness or injury associated with the service).

To monitor these areas, effective evaluative techniques, such as those described in this book, must be employed. Readers interested in accreditation and quality assurance are referred to the Further Reading list at the end of this book. It may be of interest to note that Target 31 of the WHO European targets for 'Health for All' states:

By 1990 all member states should have built effective mechanisms for ensuring the quality of patient care within their health care system.

The UK Government has accepted the aims of 'Health for All.'

Imperatives towards evaluation

Every health management team has access to extensive information about health service *activity* (e.g. bed occupancy, throughput and waiting lists), which itself is an aspect of process. Much of this is available on a daily basis. Knowledge about *outcome* is sparse. This is because outcome is inherently difficult to measure, especially in a routine manner. The difficulty in part is due to the fact that a proper assessment of outcome often requires the long-term monitoring of people after their contact with a particular sector of the health service has ceased; moreover, the gathering of usable information demands clearly defined and objective measures of outcome and their recording in a uniform manner. Despite these difficulties, there are strong market forces which are impelling those who finance health services and those who manage them to pay close attention to issues of outcome and value for money; the moves within the British National Health Service (NHS) to devolve much budgetary control, and hence accountability, to clinicians is forcing doctors and paramedicals to accept responsibility for these issues too. A detailed analysis of these market forces would be out of place here, but three important factors deserve mention as they provide a strong motivation of the evaluation of health service effectiveness.

First, there is the high pace of medical scientific advance and the commercial exploitation of this new knowledge. This has led to the introduction of many very sophisticated diagnostic devices and therapeutic machines, e.g. CAT scanners and lithotriptors. Linked to high technology in life-support systems and prostheses, there are continuing developments in the fields of transplant surgery, replacement surgery and neonatal intensive care. Pharmaceutical developments, many of them likely to be extremely expensive in practice (e.g. erythropoietin), abound. Also, developments from molecular biology and immunology are likely to have a dramatic impact on the treatment of many diseases. Secondly, the public's expectation of health services has not diminished. People want the best and if it is dramatic and highly technological then so much the better. Any notion that improved general living conditions, health promotion and disease prevention services will reduce demand for health services now seems naïve. Finally, the demographic drift towards a population with a substantially larger proportion of elderly and 'old elderly' people is producing a need for increased treatment and care of a group with multiple morbidity and high dependency levels.

While in the arena of politics there is scope for plenty of argument about the desirable level of funding of health services, one fundamental fact remains inescapable – health resources are in competition with other social requirements (e.g. education, housing, cultural activities and defence) and, in consequence, are always constrained. Unfortunately, demands for services cannot be limited by drawing a line on a governmental budget sheet. The responsibility for drawing a quart from a pint pot falls to health service managers and increasingly to clinicians.

In these circumstances, clinicians and managers are coming to realize that not all conceivable demand can be met and that choices will have to be made: choices between service developments and better criteria to decide who might most benefit from these and various existing services. This entails two things: first, the existence of far better information about the benefits accruing from services, i.e. knowledge of service effectiveness and cost-effectiveness; secondly, planning and management systems within the health service that can make optimum use of this knowledge about effectiveness. In our opinion, these two issues are inseparable and we shall discuss both later, particularly in Chapter 12.

The reforms of the NHS, though admittedly not to everybody's taste, do have one great merit. In bringing accountability to the clinicians, they force consideration of value-for-money issues. And value for money can only be sensibly addressed if we know what we are getting. So the evaluation of health service effectiveness will be a growth area.

We regard the willingness to underwrite evaluation, undertake evaluation and to use the findings of evaluation as a manifestation of a more general questioning ethic that all health professionals should share. It is sad that it has taken so long for this ethic to become prevalent. Yet, fortunately, the need for evaluation has been recognized widely and much excellent work is done in many centres. The technology of evaluation is well developed and it is upon this shared knowledge that we draw in this book.

Evaluation, as presented here, has much in common with some other important developments in health services. It ties in closely with concerns to monitor and improve the quality of services (see pp. 3–5). It links to medical and clinical audit; in particular to the kind of information that may flow from improvements in medical record-keeping and the development of clinical databases. The further development of routine information systems will bear in mind a need to satisfy some of the requirements of evaluative efforts and it is to be hoped that these systems will become less obsessed with process and pay more attention to outcome. The linking of these various systems offers exciting possibilities. However, the mere development of audit and information technologies will solve few problems unless health professionals are encouraged to think critically about their own areas of interest and are educated to handle information sensibly.

The scope of evaluation

Although evaluation will be facilitated by the developments mentioned above, it should be seen as an activity in its own right. Rarely will routine sources of information be able to answer the more complicated questions to which evaluation is addressed. This is particularly so where innovation is concerned; by definition, no routine system will be capturing information about something not in routine service. Thus the task of evaluation has to be subdivided by time, person and place. The initial evaluation of major or complicated innovation will probably take place, as it does largely at present, in specialized centres, e.g. teaching hospitals and research units. The staff involved will generally be super-specialists drawing upon support from statisticians, economists, etc. The consumers of these evaluations will be the planners, managers and clinicians at other centres. We believe it essential that these consumers be capable of looking critically at the results of such evaluation and of adapting the findings to their own circumstances. To this end, later chapters discuss some of the theoretical and methodological issues underlying 'grand' evaluation. In so doing, we do not seek to make our readers self-sufficient experts and shall refer them to other sources for greater detail. One topic we shall stress is that potential consumers of evaluative studies (e.g. managers) should be demanding that the criteria of evaluation used be sufficiently wide to encompass the concerns of those who have to implement innovation. Alternatively, the evaluators must make clear the limited relevance of the criteria they use. Thus it should not suffice for someone evaluating a new cancer therapy merely to show that tumours regress more (phase 2 clinical trial) or merely to show that survival is enhanced (phase 3 clinical trial) compared to standard therapies. We shall show that the former trial is useless for health service planning (although not for scientific purposes) and that the latter trial gives too little information. A proper evaluation, in this context, would encompass survival, quality of life, patient satisfaction, absolute cost and cost compared to alternative treatments. Only in the light of this information would management be in a position rationally to support or resist introduction of the new, and usually expensive, therapy. In so doing, they would have to adapt the findings to the likely demand at their centre and consider such matters as opportunity cost (see Chapter 5).

An evaluation that dealt with only one aspect can undoubtedly enlarge our knowledge in that small area, but 'success' in one link of the chain of events cannot be extrapolated to all others, something which enthusiastic supporters for an innovation can find very hard to resist. The customer for evaluations of health service effectiveness has to be clear about many dimensions of a service and what its widespread implication could be. This insight into the chain of events is a crucial contribution from health service managers; it is essential that they help to set the evaluation 'agenda' so that the results of the work can be related to the local structure and local resources, and so that change which may be needed can be handled i.e. *managed*, in a thoroughly professional way.

At local level, both in teaching centres and beyond, there are many other less grand but nevertheless important matters that require in-house evaluation. These may concern changes in practice or organization of services. Existing services may be modified and the outcomes monitored or new services may be introduced on a pilot basis subject to the findings of evaluation. This could pose serious problems, for at present few routinely available treatments or services have had their effectiveness quantified. Management and clinicians should react pragmatically. That is, they should recognize that evaluation is itself a costly and time-consuming process and that criteria for what should be evaluated must be agreed and that priorities need to be set on what is to be evaluated. In Chapters 3 and 12, we suggest how a core team might be constituted to assist with evaluation.

The main problem to be faced by those tackling any area thought worthy of evaluation is defining the task in a manner that makes solution feasible. We shall show by example how the goals of evaluation may be defined and how usually the task may be split into more manageable sub-tasks. At the stage of planning, a clear decision is needed about how unequivocal the findings of the evaluation need to be in order to inform decision making. The counsel of perfection is often unattainable when decisions are required quickly and at relatively little expense. While we deplore the tendency towards, quick and dirty studies, we do believe it possible to do *quick and clean*[4] work. What matters is that those doing the work fully understand the likely consequences of compromises made to facilitate rapid and cheap results and hence do not over-interpret their findings. Also, an understanding of basic theoretical and methodological principles helps avoid some not so obvious howlers.

In the next chapter, we define a number of concepts central to evaluation in preparation for putting them to use later in the book.

Chapter 2

Key concepts and the setting of objectives

Introduction

In Chapter 1, we stated our definition of evaluation. Now we shall show how the simple framework implied by that definition may be elaborated. Having an understanding of the key concepts explained here will greatly facilitate the planning of evaluative studies. We begin by exploring the idea of goals, aims and objectives and show how using these enables complicated tasks to be simplified. Then we shall explore some indices of effectiveness and finally look at some important miscellaneous topics. With this grounding completed, we shall be ready for the discussion in Chapter 3 of how to set up an evaluation.

Health service goals, aims and objectives

Understanding the concepts of goals, aims and objectives is helpful both in analysing a service prior to evaluation (indeed, the word 'goal' forms part of our definition of evaluation) and in the design of evaluative studies. We define and illustrate health service *goals*, *aims* and *objectives* as follows:

1. *Goals are the long-term, or ultimate, intent of a service.* For example, the World Health Organization 'Health for All by the Year 2000' might be a goal for our entire nation in the attainment of which the NHS has a major role to play. The goal of a health promotion service might be the elimination of 90% of lung cancer (that proportion attributable to cigarette smoking). A goal of the obstetric and paediatric services might be the total elimination of perinatal and infant morbidity. A goal of the immunization and vaccination service might be the eradication of pertussis. Often, as in 'Health for All', a goal may be a statement of ideological commitment rather than something wholly attainable in the foreseeable future; indeed, we may not at present be certain whether or how the goal can ever be attained.

2. *Aims are less ideological and more consistent with what is practicable*

now and in the short-term future. For example, health promotion services may aim for an annual reduction of 5% in the number of cigarette smokers; obstetricians might aim to give women the greatest possible choice in the mode of their delivery; the immunization and vaccination service might aim for a 95% reduction in cases of pertussis within 10 years. The achievement of aims and the formulation of new more exacting aims may be seen as stepping stones to the realization of goals.

   3. *Objectives are tasks which have to be accomplished before aims may be realized.* One aim may require the accomplishment of several tasks. For example, the control of pertussis requires (a) that efficacious vaccines be available, (b) that these are administered according to efficacious schedules, (c) that vaccines be administered to the appropriate groups in the population and (d) that vaccination uptake attain some minimum level so that herd immunity may reduce the threshold of infection and thereby indirectly reduce the risk to those who have fallen outside the vaccination net. Another example is that in order to bring about a steady reduction in the number of cigarette smokers, health promotion professionals may seek to meet the following objectives: influence government to increase tobacco taxes; influence sporting bodies to eschew tobacco sponsorship; influence local restaurants and public places to ban smoking, have greater input into the school curriculum, etc.

The difference between goals and aims is a matter of degree rather than kind, but it is often helpful to draw a distinction. Objectives, however, are different in kind from goals and aims. They are at the level of operational tasks, which have to be accomplished in order to meets aims and goals.

Thus, before embarking on an evaluative study, it is essential to understand how that study should be structured in terms of health service goals, aims and objectives. Similarly, it is essential to gain a thorough understanding of the service under examination.

Understanding a service

In seeking to understand a service, the following issues should be taken into account:

1. *Goals and aims*
   - Have these been explicitly stated? If not, can they be deduced?
2. *Theory*
   - What is the justification on current knowledge that the service can affect health outcome?
   - Do theoretical considerations suggest an optimum manner for delivery of the service?
3. *Structure*
   - What is the physical and organizational structure of the service?
   - Was this structure planned from first principles or did it evolve?
   - Who makes key decisions? For example, managers may wish to reduce

the waiting list for varicose vein surgery, but it is the consultants who decide who is to be admitted from their lists.

4. *Dynamics*
   - How does the service respond to changes in demand or need?
   - Is there any way by which those providing the service become aware of these changes?
   - How does information, both clinical and administrative, flow through the service?
   - In what manner could these factors influence effectiveness?

5. *Objectives*
   - Do the structure and dynamics of the service form a coherent whole which serves to fulfil the stated (or implied) objectives necessary for the aims and goals? (Service agreements, or contracts, can provide useful insights into what a service thinks its main objectives are.)

6. *Personalities*
   - Do all the key workers share a common notion about the goals, aims and objectives of the service?
   - How do they get on one with another? (The answer to this question may profoundly influence the range of options to be considered should changes to the service be proposed.)

Only when a service is thoroughly understood is it feasible to start planning a formal evaluation. Indeed, if during preliminary investigation it becomes obvious that the goals, aims and objectives of the service are ill-defined or that the structure and dynamics of the service are inappropriate for the aims and objectives, then further evaluation is best postponed until matters have been clarified. Moreover, the kind of detailed examination proposed here can sometimes be viewed as an evaluative process in its own right and will call upon specific techniques and skills. These matters are discussed further in Chapter 6.

Knowledge of the goals, aims and objectives of a service opens up the possibility of evaluations at one or more different levels of the service.

Levels of evaluation

While it is desirable to evaluate services in terms of achievement of goals or aims, this is not often practicable, particularly in the context of a single provider working alone and to a short time-scale. However, by consideration of the aims and objectives of a service and the manner in which these interrelate, it is usually feasible to distinguish manageable strands within what would have been a bewilderingly complicated overall evaluation. There are two techniques of simplification:

1. It may be feasible to separate aspects of a service for which individual aims and sets of objectives can be defined. In this manner, the evaluation of a service may be reduced to the piecemeal evaluation of 'sub-services'. For example, the effectiveness of a general surgical service may be tackled by

looking separately at its effectiveness for varicose vein sufferers, hernia sufferers, etc.

2. If there is good reason to believe that the meeting of the stated objectives will accomplish the avowed aims, then it will suffice to evaluate the service at the level of objectives. For example, a cervical cytology call–recall service may be evaluated in terms of the completeness and regularity of smear testing of women in the target population; this being on the (not strictly proven) assumption that some abnormal smears indicate a treatable pre-cancerous state and that the examination interval is such as to produce a sufficient yield of pre-cancerous cervices to reduce the population morbidity and mortality from cervical cancer. Thus, an evaluation of a cervical screening programme may be short-term and does not need to demonstrate reductions in population cervical cancer morbidity.

We suggest that health service evaluation be approached in a *pragmatic* manner. Go for that which is feasible, for that which you feel confident of tackling and succeeding in, and for that where the likely pay-off is worthwhile. Your knowledge of the principles (theory) underlying the service and of its practical realization (structure, dynamics and personalities) will direct you to those aspects (objectives) of the service which are crucial for the overall effectiveness of the service.

Study goals, aims and objectives

These are analogous to the service goals, aims and objectives mentioned earlier in the chapter. Ideally, there should within a unit, district or region be clearly defined goals for a programme of health service evaluation. This programme will consist of a series of carefully designed studies, each of which should have clearly defined aims. In order to meet those aims, a set of objectives must be fulfilled during the investigation. Thinking about a task in this manner makes it much easier to design the investigation and the writing of a study protocol will dispel vague ideas (see Chapter 3).

In general, the fewer aims the better: multiple aims tend to lead to elaborate studies which may fail. Also, simplicity of intent and design usually leads to simplicity of analysis and interpretation. Thus an investigation programme may have multiple goals and aims but a single study should not.

Choosing study objectives

The key element of any study of effectiveness is *the comparison between actual practice and some standard*. The standard may be absolute (e.g. the explicitly stated aims of the service) or comparative (e.g. the achievement of a differently organized service of the same intent). In general, in the context of unit- or district-based research, *it will not be feasible to evaluate directly in terms of morbidity or mortality outcomes* – this statement will be justified in Chapter 11 where the statistical issues of study size and power are discussed. Moreover, in small-scale research, it is often impracticable to look for changes in intermediate outcomes such as the distribution of birth weights following, say, some social support intervention in the care of 'disadvantaged' pregnant women. Nevertheless, investigators can usually create study objectives which lead to the examination of service objectives known, or believed, directly to influence health outcome, e.g. vaccination uptake, cervical screening uptake, waiting time for artificial hip replacement, etc.

Indices of effectiveness

In our definition of the evaluation of service effectiveness and at several other points in the preceding discussion, we have stressed that the ultimate goal is to assess the *outcome* or impact of health services on the population. Also, we have shown how when this goal is not directly attainable, it may often be approached through proxy measures or through the evaluation of intermediate processes necessary for effectiveness to be realized. At this point, it is desirable to examine some concepts and indices which pertain to effectiveness.

Efficacy

A clinical service cannot attain its goals unless its component parts and the way these relate one to another, and the manner which the service is targeted to the community, are themselves effective (in the general usage of the word). The component parts may comprise an array of diagnostic, treatment or caring procedures: these must themselves be efficacious if the entire service is to be effective. A procedure may, loosely, be said to be efficacious if on average it has a clearly demonstrated beneficial effect on prognosis or suffering. The structure, organizational efficiency and targeting of the service determine whether procedures known to be efficacious on selected individuals (often in ideal circumstances) will give such benefit to appropriate members of the general community.

Measures of efficacy are statistical in nature because they pertain to changes in prognosis, which is itself a statistical concept. Thus, findings from studies of efficacy tend to be summarized in terms of proportions of patients improving or in remission after defined periods of time. When death is at issue, the results are presented as survival curves or, more crudely, as the proportion alive after 1 year, five years, etc.

In general, the best way to determine efficacy is through well-constructed clinical trials. Indeed, the theory and practice of clinical trials is, perhaps, the most strongly developed field within health service evaluation. There is a variety of techniques and well-developed statistical theory to aid in their analysis. Nevertheless, clinical trials are too frequently badly done and very often when conducted in a methodologically sound manner they neglect to address issues pertinent to service planning. Clinical trials are discussed further in Chapter 7.

Efficiency

This is about *organization*, i.e. the internal day-to-day running of health services. It can simply be a matter of comparing 'inputs' with 'outputs', assuming that an efficient service has more outputs for given inputs than a less efficient service; for example, a higher number of patients treated in a lower number of beds. However, in the health service, it can also be argued that the service is only efficient if it is also effective, because otherwise the resources are wasted; all the patients may need to come back into hospital if their treatment is not effective.

The distinction between efficiency and effectiveness is as follows: a service is efficient if it does what it does well; it is effective if it produces benefit. A service may be effective and inefficient or vice versa, more frequently the latter.

Cost-effectiveness

Cost-effectiveness is the financial cost for a given outcome. Examination of the cost-effectiveness of a service relates the total cost of the service to its impact on the community. Different versions of a service having the same objectives may be conceivable (they may differ in the procedures on offer or in structure and delivery); sensible health service planners will choose the cheapest version which delivers the required impact in a manner acceptable to the community. The cost-effectiveness of an existing service may be enhanced by improving its efficiency or its effectiveness. Cost-effectiveness analyses usually consider only health service costs; also, they are difficult to interpret if there is more than one plausible measure of outcome.

Cost-utility

'Utility' is a concept of economic theory which attempts to provide a common measure of the satisfaction derived from all consumption. A utility, or value, may be attached to the expected outcome of a treatment or service. One such utility measure is 'Quality Adjusted Life Years' (QALYs). It consists of the average expectation of life following treatment, multiplied by an index of quality of life. The index of quality is a weighted average of a set of scores each of which represents an aspect of life-quality (e.g. pain) during the years remaining to typical patients; thus survival in a comatose condition for 5 years would score considerably lower than restoration to near normal function for 3 years. Division of the average total cost of treatment and care by the QALYs gives rise to the cost per quality adjusted life year (an example of a cost-utility measure); it then becomes possible to compare treatments for the same disease in terms of cost per QALY gained by one treatment over the other. Also, cost per QALY may be compared among treatments for diverse conditions, e.g.

artificial hip replacement vs renal transplant. It should be obvious from this brief account that many assumptions underlie the use of cost-utility analysis and also that the QALY concept is most easily applicable when expectation of life is an important outcome measure.

Cost–benefit

Cost–benefit analysis attempts to measure all the inputs and outputs of treatment and care in common units, usually money (pounds sterling, US dollars, etc.). It thus becomes possible to compare treatments or entire health programmes for the same or differing health problems. The 'cost' element encompasses the obvious financial costs of treatment and care and also wider costs to the patient, his family and society at large; these wider costs include loss of earnings, state benefits, disruption of family life, and loss of function through side-effects of treatment and sequelae of disease. 'Benefits' include restoration of function to the patient and any consequent ability of the patient and his or her family to contribute to the common good, e.g. by being in employment. Some costs and benefits are naturally measurable on a monetary scale, but for others the translation to money-equivalents may be controversial.

The results of cost–benefit analyses may be presented either as the net benefit, i.e. benefit minus cost, or as the ratio of cost to benefit. The net benefit provides a measure of the *absolute* benefit to society of a health care programme; this could be an overall loss. When comparing cost–benefit analyses for different health care programmes, care must be taken to ensure not only that the monetary translations of costs and benefits are acceptable but also that the ranges of costs and benefits considered in different studies are sufficiently similar and far-reaching.

Cost-effectiveness, cost–benefit and cost-utility are also covered in Chapter 5.

Quality of care

Maxwell[1] has suggested six aspects to quality of care: access to services, relevance to need for the whole community, equity, social acceptability, effectiveness, efficiency and economy. It should not be assumed that these can be independently assessed. Thus, we suggest that the evaluation of health service effectiveness should be seen as part of a wider concern for quality of care. Nevertheless, within this wide remit it is prudent to look separately at effectiveness issues because to do so entails standing aside from the day-to-day provision of care, whereas much that is done specifically to promote quality (e.g. quality circles, medical audit and nursing audit) is at the level of the individual patient contact. However, we acknowledge an overlap and shall discuss medical/clinical audit in Chapter 4.

Lurking ideologies

An ideological stance is implicit in every attempt to evaluate health services and distribute health care resources. Investigators of service effectiveness should try to make plain the ideological assumptions which lead to the perception of need for a particular study and which inevitably will influence the choice of study aims and objectives. Even what appear to be merely techniques, such as cost-effectiveness, cost-utility and cost–benefit analysis, contain an implicit ideology; depending on circumstances, this ideology may or may not be acceptable. In our more detailed examination of some of these concepts, we shall try to draw out implicit assumptions and leave our readers to make up their own minds about them.

It can be tempting to confuse *ideology* with overt political dogma; individuals claim that they are 'non-political' because they are not signed up members of a 'large P' political party. However, we all have a different way of looking at life; nobody is purely disinterested. The importance of recognizing this for evaluating service effectiveness is that different approaches to an evaluative study can lead to different conclusions, each of which may be entirely valid, but where it is the underlying ideology, not the evaluative technique *per se*, which produces the result. The danger lies in not acknowledging this. The role of ideology in decision making is discussed in Chapter 12.

Chapter 3

Planning and executing health service evaluation

Introduction

Thinking in detail about planning and executing an evaluation study may, at first sight, appear constraining and bureaucratic, but consider our advice to be like a suggestion that you read the map before embarking on a journey to a somewhat vague destination. Map reading can be done at various points along the way, but an initial scan of the distance, key stopping points and main routes should help the trip to be accomplished more safely, with less time wasting and less frustration. You may be able to appreciate more the value of your companions along the way and not run out of petrol in embarrassing or difficult places.

Apportioning responsibility

Any initiative which goes beyond the current routine tasks of district management will require careful planning, appropriate resources and a recognized place in the management structure.

Ideas for service evaluation will come from a number of sources: health authority members, service providers, managers, complainants and others. If an evaluative study is set up, there will a core set of tasks which are better managed if they are clearly identified and allocated to named individuals. These tasks are:

1. *Commissioning the study and requiring intelligible reports.* An individual or group will have to take the explicit responsibility of choosing an evaluative study. This responsibility also extends to having a clear idea of how to use the results of the study, and what arrangements are in hand to be kept in touch with all relevant events. This should usually be on the basis of exception reporting; more detailed involvement is the responsibility of the overseer.

2. *Overseeing the study.* Here the responsibility is making sure that the

study happens as intended, that information is being collected, the right people consulted, the right reports produced for the right people at the right time in the right place, and that there are no diversions from the original intention unless these can be stringently justified. The allocation of resources for the study is also part of the overseer's responsibility.

3. *Doing the study.* Here the responsibilities involve reviewing the literature, planning the study, establishing communications and writing reports. It is essential – but often forgotten – to be clear about who has prime responsibility for doing the research, and how much of their time should be spent on this rather than other activities.

4. *Supporting and enabling.* Resources are required, as are help and participation from a variety of people. The supporters/enablers may provide assistance for the research task itself (e.g. clerical support), or they may be service providers whose service is being provided. The overseers should ensure that there is adequate support for the 'doer' to achieve the aims of the study in the time intended.

The resulting hierarchy is set out below. It is important to agree this at the beginning of any study in order to avoid two common failings of health service evaluation that are more likely to occur if the process is not properly managed, i.e. it may never be finished or, if finished, it will have nowhere to go.

The Evaluation Hierarchy
Commissioner (an individual or group)
Overseer (often better as multidisciplinary group)
Doer (often an individual)
Supporters/enablers (many different individuals)

Whatever structural solution is adopted, it will be necessary for named individuals to accept responsibility for overseeing and undertaking evaluation tasks. That is, there should be some kind of evaluation team with effective leadership.

Resources

Unless health authorities are in the unlikely position of being able to employ people specifically to supervise evaluation studies, it will be necessary to divert some skilled senior staff from other tasks. These staff will require the following resources:

1. *Time.* The in-house resources used for health service evaluation are often invisible because they simply involve a diversion of existing resources from one task to another. The key element is time, and it needs to be clearly allocated at all levels in the responsible hierarchy. Reading around a topic is time-consuming. So is writing an intelligible report on the basis of that reading and any data which have been collected. Senior managers are aware of this and

have a responsibility to ensure that their less experienced colleagues are not forced to learn this the painful and unproductive way.

2. *Library.* The importance of reading literature on a given topic cannot be overestimated. Helpful librarians, who guide researchers who cannot see the wood for the trees, are worth their weight in gold.

3. *Secretarial and clerical.* This can extend to assisting in literature searches, keeping in touch with participants, recording key data, making copies of everything, making appointments, taking messages, etc. There are also the additional costs of stationery, postage, 'phones, faxing and photocopying – these are all needed, and failure to acknowledge them explicitly could ruin an otherwise superb initiative.

4. *Fieldworkers.* Fieldwork, which is often short-term, may be under-taken by administrative assistants with the agreement of unit managers (indeed, this is excellent general experience for them). Enthusiasm and commitment are highly desirable, but may also need to be supplemented by training, for example in interviewing. Professional interviewers can be expensive, but are often sufficiently efficient and effective to make the additional costs worthwhile in terms of time and effort saved, and because the results are reproducible and of high quality.

5. *Statistical advice.* This should be obtained at the beginning of the study when it is being designed, and not just at the end, when there is a huge barrow load of data with no means of sorting or interpreting it.

6. *Information advice.* Find out what is already collected and / or available before embarking on the collection of yet more primary data.

7. *Computing advice.* This is not the same as either statistical advice or information advice: statistical advice will help the researcher understand what numbers of people or tests need to be included in a study, and how to analyse the results; information advice covers routinely available information like performance indicators, hospital costing returns and so forth. Computing advice, however, covers the technology which is appropriate to the sort of study you are undertaking, i.e. the sort of machine (hardware) and the sort of data processing (software) which may be required or are available.

Selection of services to be evaluated

The process of selection of the services to be evaluated is largely the responsibility of the research commissioner. There are usually three main criteria involved:

1. *Political feasibility.* It is essential for the evaluation team to gain confidence from some early successes; thus, initially, services should be chosen where goodwill and cooperation are likely. Some people may find the notion of evaluating service effectiveness personally threatening or just a worthless distraction from matters they regard as more important.

Political feasibility does not detract from the scientific rigour or usefulness of the study. Inexperienced researchers tend to feel that the only 'worthwhile' type of service evaluation is that which is immensely complicated, time-consuming and challenging. However, well-defined studies that are successfully completed and used by the service in question are of far more benefit to evaluators and to the service as a whole. And beware, superficially 'easy' situations politically may conceal immense interpersonal undercurrents and complexities. Take nothing for granted.

2. *Urgency/feasibility of change.* Obviously, initial attention should be directed towards services where there is doubt about their effectiveness and where it might be feasible to effect change. The effectiveness of the service may be challenged by patients, the Community Health Council, authority members or health service professionals. Before an evaluation is commissioned, information will be required as to:

- the precise nature of the challenge;
- whether the challenge is an isolated event or consistent with reports from other sources (formal or informal); and
- what the covert objectives of the complainant/challenger are thought to be.

A judgement can then be made as to whether an evaluation should be commissioned, how it should be managed, and who should do it and how.

3. *Technical feasibility.* Essentially, this is what you think may be accomplished in the stipulated time-scale with the available resources. This is strongly dependent upon the chosen objectives of the evaluation, which in turn determine the outcome measures to be used in estimating service effectiveness. It is worth remembering that it is better to do a small study thoroughly, and be able to follow through the implications, rather than be overwhelmed by an ambitious project which cannot be completed.

Time-scale

Evaluations of service effectiveness have to be credible. This requires careful background reading, a high standard of data collection and a report that is sufficiently well written for readers to use the information. All these processes take time, and it is generally better to overestimate the time required and deliver a report early, than the other way round.

A project to be completed in 9 months will probably break down as follows:

- 2 months preparation;
- 5 months data collection; and
- 2 months data analysis, interpretation, writing up and presentation.

Make allowance for holiday months.

The most common problems are underestimates of the time it takes to do a thorough preparation, and the time it takes to extract the salient features from a mass of data and reports. Intelligent preparation not only provides a secure grounding for subsequent data collection, but may indicate that there is little more to be gained from further research – there is already enough information to guide local decisions. Good report writing is a skill few of us possess and, consequently, enough time should be allowed to draft and redraft and decide the key messages to be conveyed in any final report. From the beginning of a project, it will be useful to set target dates to ensure that each stage is completed on time.

Planning the study

There are six key phases involved in planning a study. They tend to form a critical path, as set out in Fig. 3.1, where each phase relies on the completion of at least one other before it can begin. In other words, designing a study cannot be done until the objectives have been clarified. Also, the means of data collection rely critically on the study design. However, writing the protocol, and establishing channels of communication, should go on throughout.

Fig. 3.1 Key phases in planning a study

Critical point / Phase (see text)	Setting objectives	Selecting study design	Organizing data collection	Protocol	Setting up channels of communication
(A) Background information	●	●			●
(B) Setting objectives		●	●	●	●
(C) Select design			●	●	●
(D) Data collection				●	●
(E) Protocol				●	●
(F) Channels of communication				●	●

The work of planning the study may be the responsibility of the 'doer'. A clear mechanism should be agreed for that individual to report back through the hierarchy ('overseer' and 'commissioner') described earlier. The process of planning the study should simultaneously enlist the help of those people needed to participate as enablers or supporters, e.g. direct care providers.

The details of each phase of planning the study are given below.

Phase A: Gathering background information

This exercise serves two purposes: first, it will help you understand the service and, secondly, it will provide ideas as to what comparisons should provide the basis for your study. Once a service has been chosen for study, the following steps and questions should be considered:

1. Gain a thorough knowledge of the structure and dynamics of the service. It also helps to know something of the personalities involved.
2. Are the goals of the service explicitly stated?
3. Was the service planned or did it just evolve, i.e. has the structure ever been carefully thought out?
4. What is known about the composition of the population being served, e.g. size, age structure, projected size and age structure, geographical dispersion? These data are often available from routine sources (see Chapter 4).
5. What is known about relevant mortality and morbidity among the population being served?
6. What is known from the literature about the efficacy of the treatments and technologies being used in the service? Are these, on the basis of current knowledge, the most appropriate?
7. What is known from the literature about the effectiveness of similar services elsewhere?
8. Are there services with similar goals but organized substantially differently from yours? Can anything be learned from these?
9. How has the effectiveness of these services been tested elsewhere? Can those methods be adapted for local use?
10. What is known about the efficiency of the local service? This information may be gained from performance indicators (see Chapter 4), and comparisons with other districts across the country are easily made.

Only armed with background knowledge and a specific understanding of the particular service will it be possible to pose questions for an evaluation. It may also save a great deal of trouble later.

Phase B: Setting objectives

Evaluation is concerned with assessing whether or not a service achieves its goals. The evaluation of effectiveness is characterized by an interest in those goals which relate to outcome, i.e. the impact of the service on the well-being of individual patients and the community. In Chapter 2, there is further discussion of these matters and of the concepts involved. The following factors determine the effectiveness of a service:

1. Efficacy of individual diagnostic, preventive, treatment or caring procedures employed by the service, i.e. do they work?
2. Correct targeting of the service, i.e. do those people most in need of the service get it?
3. Acceptability of the service to the community and satisfaction of individual clients.
4. Ease of access to the service, e.g. time and distance of travel, and mode of referral.
5. Whether the structure of the service (e.g. treatment schedules, equipment and staffing) has a bearing on outcome.
6. Efficiency of the service, i.e. is it managed in a manner which makes best use of existing resources?

Any evaluation of a service must involve comparison of that service, or of the result of a change to the service, with some standard. Thus the key task in planning a study is the selection of suitable indices of comparison. The choice of these will depend upon the goals being evaluated. The objectives are a specific statement of what will be measured and how it will be compared.

Phase C: Selecting study designs

The choice of study design is determined by the following factors:

1. The aims of the study and the precise objectives which have to be met to fulfil those aims.
2. The time-scale and resources for the study.
3. The degree to which 'scientific rigour' is desired, e.g. is the study intended merely to aid internal district 'seat of the pants' planning or is it intended that the results be applicable elsewhere?

Several important types of study design are discussed in Chapters 6, 7 and 8. Broadly speaking, the sort of study which may be felt to be most appropriate can be a description based on testimony, or an analysis of historical or cross-sectional data, or an intervention study, or a patient satisfaction survey or a controlled trial. It is most important that you are happy with the approach you are taking and feel you understand it rather than aiming for a counsel of perfection which may not be achievable.

Phase D: Organizing data collection

We recommend that the following advice be borne in mind when the organization of data collection is being considered:

1. Plan to record only those data which are necessary for the study objectives.

Decide in advance how the information/statistics are to be dealt with during analysis. That is, while planning you should consider exactly how each item of information will be used and how it will contribute to the final conclusion. This implies that if a study is investigating well-posed questions, then the range of possible answers and actions to flow from them will have been anticipated. Thus if numerical data are to be collected, it can be helpful to draw up outline tables of how the results will appear when presented.

2. Decide how the data are to be collected, i.e. by whom, when and where.
3. Decide how the data are to be checked and who is to be responsible for this. It is much easier to correct data near the time of collection than at the end of the study.
4. Decide how the data are to be stored. For simple studies, it may suffice to analyse data manually from written records.
5. If it is anticipated that a computer will be required to aid in the analysis, then seek advice during the planning phase of the study on coding and storage (see pp. 154–7). Make sure that the necessary technical expertise will be available during the analysis phase.
6. If information about individuals is to be recorded on a computer file, it may be necessary to register under the Data Protection Act (1984). This Act is complicated and advice should be taken. The Act covers data stored on all electronic devices including microcomputers. All districts should have a data protection officer.

Phase E: The protocol

A written protocol is an essential document in any study. Its principal purpose is to help you clarify your own thoughts, but it can also be a useful way of describing to others exactly what the study is about. It should contain:

1. A brief statement of the background to the study, i.e. the context in which it takes place.
2. A precise statement of the aims and objectives (think of aims as strategy and objectives as tactics).
3. Details of the study design.
4. Details of proposed data collection, quality control, recording and processing.
5. Where applicable, details of how confidentiality will be maintained. Public health physicians should accept responsibility for the safe keeping and proper use of clinical data about individual patients. Arrangements may need to be made to register under the Data Protection Act (1984) because of computer files with information about individuals.
6. An outline of how the analysis will be tackled.
7. A timetable for the study from initial data collection to presentation of results.
8. A clear statement of who is responsible for each aspect of the study.

9. An estimate of the resources required: person time and skill level for data collection, clerical tasks, analysis, etc.; equipment; consumables, etc.

The protocol will go through several stages of drafting as the investigators clarify their ideas about the study. It could form the basis of a contract between an investigating team and those to whom they are answerable. If, subsequently, there are any disagreements about the objectives or execution of the study, the protocol may be referred to as the authoritative source.

The draft protocol will often be improved by discussing it with the key players in the study (see next section). A benefit of sharing the written protocol is that participation of the key players in the evolution of the protocol is likely to help secure their commitment and understanding.

Phase F: Channels of communication

Before data collection starts, all of those upon whom cooperation depends must be conversant with the nature of the project and have given it their support. This can be a time-consuming exercise but it is worthwhile in the long run. Studies may founder because insufficient attention has been paid to the importance of communication, or people may withdraw goodwill from further studies if they feel that they have been used in an inappropriate manner. Developing the protocol with their help is a useful means of taking this forward.

When planning a project, draw up a list of people who need to know or whom it would be courteous to inform. Put by each person's name a comment as to whether that person is likely to be supportive or not. If the latter, try to analyse the reason and consider how support may be obtained from that person.

The following may need to be considered:

- chief executive and other senior managers, both general and unit;
- ethical committee;
- chairmen of divisions involved;
- consultants must be involved if their patients are being investigated;
- nursing staff must be consulted if their wards are involved;
- medical records officer;
- clinic clerks;
- local medical committee; and
- general practitioners and the FHSA if the study is general practice-based or entails contacting patients on GP lists.

This is by no means a complete checklist; for instance, it may be necessary to consult or inform trades union representatives.

The protocol is a useful document to show such people. Consider whether the district management board, unit management boards, clinical directors or district medical advisory committee need to know.

Piloting the study

The pilot study is a 'trial run' undertaken before embarking on a full-scale project. The purposes of the pilot include:

- confirming that the study management hierarchy is aware of its responsibilities;
- checking that the selected method/study design is appropriate for the data to be collected;
- confirming the political/technical feasibility of the study; and
- checking that the time-scale is reasonable.

Only after this trial run has been completed will it be possible to be sure that the whole study will work. Pilot studies are a thoroughly practical means of assessing, for example:

- whether the field workers are sufficiently trained;
- how long a questionnaire really does take to complete;
- whether the answers and questions make sense;
- whether the setting (e.g. the out-patient clinic or the ward) really can be used as planned;
- whether there are other people who should be informed;
- whether participants are as available and willing as thought; and
- whether data can be analysed as intended.

Time spent on a pilot study is never wasted. If the study plan needs no amendment, then the research can go ahead; if changes are required, then they can be made before too much time and effort is expended.

Carrying out the study

With so much care taken on the preparation and communication, it may feel as though the study should virtually do itself. However, it may be useful to consider the following additional issues:

1. It is often courteous to display notices informing people that a study is in progress, describing its aims and objectives.
2. Researchers or interviewers should have a clear and official identification.
3. Participants should be provided with an address or 'phone number where they can contact the research commissioner in the event they have a complaint or a comment.
4. All fieldworkers must thoroughly understand and, if necessary, be trained in their tasks before data collection commences.
5. The team leader ('doer') must keep a firm grip on the study; he or she must ensure at all times that the investigators do not deviate from the agreed protocol.
6. The team leader must personally supervise the quality control of the data

being collected; he or she must keep in daily touch with all aspects of the study and all members of the team.

7. Problems and unanticipated events are bound to occur; the team leader must act decisively and be prepared to jettison some of the aims if this is necessary to preserve the bulk of the study.

It is a nice touch to write and thank everyone who is involved after the study has been completed.

Analysis of information

The study plan and research protocol should have already identified how data will be analysed. The following hints may also be useful:

1. Use simple methods when examining the data, e.g. tabulations, graphs and charts.
2. Look for substantial differences or changes, i.e. changes which in practical terms are clearly interesting and potentially important.
3. Look for consistency among the data; several criteria of effectiveness showing improvement are far more convincing than a conflicting pattern of change.
4. Do not become obsessed with statistical significance; consistency and plausibility of results are far more important (see pp. 169–78).
5. Use only techniques you fully understand. Beware particularly of computer analysis packages which offer esoteric analyses – these may not be appropriate to your data.
6. Do not allow anyone to start an analysis on a computer until the data have been thoroughly checked for errors.
7. Be aware that lack of apparent change does not establish that there has been no change; the study may have been too small to 'prove' anything, but still may describe, very importantly, the way a service is going.
8. Think carefully of any extraneous factors which may have affected the result. Could this effect have been to give a false impression of change when none existed or could it have diminished real change?

Presentation of results

The purpose of presenting the results is to guide the reader or audience through the process of the research, and to interpret some of the most important analyses. Pages of tables are of little use to most readers. It is often useful when describing the results of the study, to ask oneself 'so what?' – and supply an answer.

Bear the following points in mind:

1. A good presentation will be intelligible to the audience for whom it is intended.

2. The main findings should be emphasized, inessential details should be omitted or relegated to appendices.
3. The readers should be able to check for themselves the main gist of the findings from simply presented tables, graphs or charts. Complicated analytical techniques, if used, should merely bring out fine detail and an understanding of them should not be essential to a critical assessment of the import of the findings.
4. Use unpretentious language.
5. Define all technical terms.
6. Explain the practical meaning of unfamiliar concepts (illustrating with examples can be helpful).
7. Present a summary of the study and its findings at the beginning of the report – some people only read summaries.
8. State the background to the study and its aims, i.e. why the study took place.
9. State the principal conclusions.
10. State the options for action to flow from these conclusions.
11. Have a draft of the report assessed by a person of similar background to the intended readership before you publish.
12. If you are making a 'live' presentation, do rehearse it beforehand in front of a colleague.
13. Keep it short.

In conclusion, results from which no action flows are worthless. The range of legitimate actions includes doing nothing further, but this must be an act of volition and not merely a consequence of apathy. Those actively involved in an evaluation of effectiveness are, through their intimate knowledge of the subject matter, often the best placed to act as advocates for change; also, they can draw lessons from the experience which may suggest further avenues of fruitful enquiry. Whether improvement of services will flow from evaluations of effectiveness depends partly on the power of this advocacy and partly on whether the advocates have a place high enough in the management structure to demand attention. These matters are taken further in Chapter 12.

Chapter 4

Using routinely gathered data to assist in evaluation

Introduction

The benefits and problems with using routine data for evaluative purposes will be discussed. The NHS produces large amounts of data routinely. The advantages of using routine data for evaluation are:

- the data are readily available;
- no extra or visible cost is involved in their collection; and
- time trend studies are easy to perform as routine data are updated at set intervals of time.

The disadvantages of using routine data are:

- because they were not specifically designed for the evaluative purpose, they might not meet all the requirements;
- the data may be inaccurate; and
- the data may be out of date.

Note also that difficulties sometimes occur when trying to link local health authority information with local authority information; these arise because the boundaries of these authorities are sometimes not co-terminus.

As an example of problems associated with routine data, one can consider the precursor of the Korner data sets, namely Hospital Activity Analysis (HAA). It was well recognized that information from this source was often inaccurate and many years out of date. For these reasons, consultants were rightly sceptical of the data and dialogue between managers and doctors was often impeded by the lack of robustness of the data.

It has been suggested[1] that the NHS can be considered to deal with the contents of three boxes. The largest box contains the community at large, for instance the population served by a district health authority. Some of the members of this box may, however, become ill and visit their GP, and thus a subset of the main population is patients actively receiving attention from GP practices. A small percentage of this population will be referred to hospital and will form the major part of the hospital population (the hospital will also receive some patients directly from the district population through the accident and emergency department).

For information purposes, this three-box approach is useful as routine information is available on the district as a whole (the largest box), on the GP practice population (a smaller box) and on the hospital population (the smallest box). The relationship between these boxes is illustrated in Fig. 4.1.

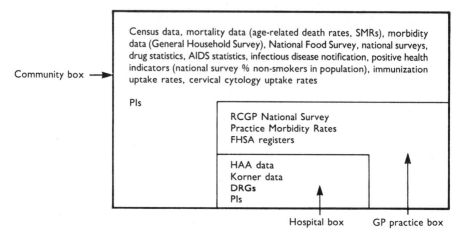

Fig. 4.1   Some data available in the community, GP practice and hospital boxes.

It is a sad reflection on our information systems that the amount of routine information available is inversely related to the size of the population in the three boxes. This is possibly related to the fact that the NHS is finance-driven and not epidemiologically-driven; hospitals are more expensive and hence more information is required of them.

The analysis of organizations in terms of structure, process and outcome has been mentioned in Chapter 1; routine information is available in relation to all three in the NHS, but it is sparse with respect to outcome.

The community box

The census

The census provides data about the structure of the population and is a useful source of denominator data. The first census was undertaken in the UK in 1801, and with the sole exception of 1941 a census has been undertaken every 10 years since then. An information industry has grown around the census. David Rhind, editor of the *Census User's Handbook*,[2] makes the following statement:

> The Census of Population is certainly a major decennial event in Britain: the taking of the 1981 census involved the employment of more than

129,000 people, cost about £45 million and was designed to elicit information from every one of the twenty million or so households in this country. The enterprise of taking the Census contained individual elements of both tragedy and humour: in Northern Ireland, a census enumerator was shot dead as she collected the census forms while, on a lighter note Mrs Beatrice Smith of Weymouth sent a bill for £5 to the Secretary of State for Social Services for the seventy minutes she devoted to completing the census questionnaire. OPCS received no less than 18,000 telephone calls from enumerators and the public over the few days around census night, covering a vast range of queries from the absurd to the arcane.

The above excerpt illustrates the complexity of the task. The most recent census was in April 1991. The next census is due in 2001.

The basic building block for the census is the enumeration district (ED; see Fig. 4.2). Each ED is serviced by one enumerator who delivers and collects the census forms from each household within the ED. The average population of an ED is about 500 in an urban area and about 150 in a rural area. In the 1981 census, there were about 110,000 EDs in England and Wales. The totality of EDs cover the country without overlap or omission.

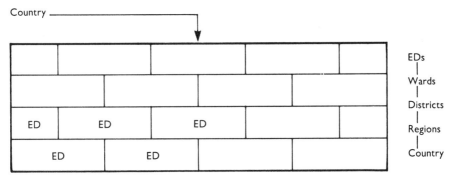

Fig. 4.2   The national census represented by the wall can be considered to be built up from building blocks of census information from enumerated districts. Small aggregations of EDS form wards, wards are aggregated to districts and districts are aggregated to regions.

Data obtained from EDs form the basis for small area statistics (SAS). Unfortunately, EDs may change from census to census so that small area statistics comparisons over time are not always possible. The Office of Population, Census and Surveys (OPCS) are aware of this problem and made arrangements for some small area consistency between the 1971 and 1981 censuses. Such comparable areas are known as census tracts. A tract can be as small as an individual ED or comprise a group of EDs. For each local government district, data are available from OPCS on census tracts for that district. ED data can be aggregated at ward or local district level or higher. Also, national, district and ward level data can be obtained from OPCS. Difficulties arise if health authority and local government boundaries are not contiguous. The advent of computer-mapping facilities with digitized boundaries for local authorities and health authorities has eased this problem and enabled the more efficient matching of data between these two authorities to take place.

The contents of the census varies from census to census but normally contains personal details of the head of the household (e.g. name, age and sex) and details of other people present in the household on census night. Details will also be required of educational qualifications, occupation and country of birth as well as details relating to physical accommodation, e.g. type of accommodation (rented or owner-occupied), facilities within the accommodation and car ownership.

From the census the age and sex structure of the population can be obtained as well as the social and ethnic class structure. Such information is of importance when defining the health needs of the population. One of the major tasks of health authorities in future will be to define the health needs of their population so that contracts can be drawn up with provider organizations to meet these. The OPCS longitudinal study (see below) will be one source of data linking age and health.

The OPCS longitudinal study

The longitudinal study (LS) is based on a 1% sample of the resident population of England and Wales. It brings together information about these people from the 1971, 1981 and 1991 censuses and from the registration of births and deaths, cancer registrations and from migration as recorded at the National Health Service Central Register. In 1990, an LS user manual was published; it serves as a useful source of reference (see Appendix A).

Population estimates

Census data rapidly become out of date due to births and deaths in the population and migration. Using data from a variety of sources, OPCS annually prepares population estimates for that inter-census year. For any particular year, the first estimates to be made are the national ones, followed by local authority and NHS authority to district level. It should be borne in mind that some local authorities make their own inter-census year estimates of population; these take account of local knowledge about the movement of population and the use of housing stock. Thus, the populations used by local authorities and the health service for planning purposes may differ even though they relate to the same geographically defined population.

Population projection

Population projections for the UK by sex and age have been made since the 1920s. Originally, they were used in connection with long-term financial estimates for social insurance and pension planning. Regional population projections were produced in the 1960s and since then projections at sub-regional level (e.g. district) have become available. Such projections are widely used for planning purposes and serve as the denominator for the calculation of many rates.

The demographic component method is used in calculating population projections. Starting from a base population (the census year population), assumptions are made about future birth rates, death rates and migration rates. Births will swell a population, deaths will lower it and migration – depending on whether it is into or out of an area – could enhance or diminish it. Of these three factors, death rates are the easiest to estimate in the medium to short-term. Future birth rates can swing dramatically depending on economic, social and political changes affecting the community. Net migration flows are also affected by such factors. At the sub-national level, migration is usually the main cause of population change and, due to the lack of comprehensive statistics, internal migration is hard to estimate. Labour Force Surveys and the National Health Service Central Register – from which migration into and out of GPs' lists can be obtained – are two sources of data for estimating migration rates.

Congenital abnormalities and disability

OPCS holds a register of congenital malformations; statistics for district health authorities are regularly published. Many local authorities and district health authorities have disability or handicap registers. Education departments have a list of children who have been assessed under the 1981 Education Act as having special educational needs. Nationally, there is an OPCS study of disability. The study shows that the prevalence of disability was 21 per 1000 children in the age range 0–4 years, 38 per 1000 aged 5–9 years, and 35 per 1000 age 10–15 years.

Acorn

Commercial organizations have used census data to produce saleable information for marketing purposes. CACI Inc. has produced Acorn (A Classification of Residential Neighbourhoods). Marketing organizations tend to use such data. It can also be used as an indicator of socio-economic disparity. For the Acorn system, 40 key census variables that covered demographic housing and socio-economic variables were extracted from the census for each of about 120,000 census enumeration districts in the UK. A cluster analysis was then performed on the census enumeration districts on the basis of their performance against the 40 key variables. Thirty-six types of residential neighbourhoods were identified, which are often aggregated into 11 neighbourhood groups.

Other sources of data which could be used as denominator data are shown in Table 4.1, which lists the frequency of the routine survey, the sample frame, respondents contacted, the sample size and approximate response ratio.

Table 4.1   Some routine surveys

Survey	Sample frame	Frequency	Type respondent	Sample size	Response ratio (%)
Census	Detailed local inspection	10 years	Household head	Full count	100
General Household	Electoral register	Continuous	Household	15,000	~ 80
Family Expenditure	Electoral register	Continuous	Household	11,000	~ 70
National Food	Electoral register	Continuous	Household	13,750	~ 60
Labour Force	Electoral register	Quarterly	Household	15,000 plus boost 44,000 March–May	~ 85
National Dwelling	Valuation list	*ad hoc*	Household	375,000	~ 85
European Community Consumer Attitude	Electoral register	4 monthly	Household head	6445	~ 75

Composite measures of deprivation

Composite indices based on the census have been developed. These entail combining a number of presumed indicators of need or relative deprivation into a single score. These scores are then computed for various populations (e.g. districts and electoral wards) and can be used as a guide to where need for additional health or social resources might be greatest. However, before taking such scoring systems at face value, read pp. 152–4. Two commonly used ones are UPA8 and the Townsend Index.

UPA8: The Jarman Underprivileged Area Source

A national survey asked GPs to list the relative contribution of certain census variables to their workload. Based on this survey, UPA8 was developed. It consists of eight variables, hence UPA8. The variables and their weights are shown in Table 4.2.

Before variables are combined to form the UPA8 index, they are transformed to try and normalize variable distribution; normalization entails placing the variables on a common scale and making their frequency distributions more nearly symmetrical. It should be noted that the variables have different weights. These reflect the GPs' views on the relative workloads

Table 4.2 Variables used in the Jarman Score

Variable	Weight
% elderly living alone	6.62
% aged under 5	4.64
% social class V	3.74
% unemployed	3.34
% one-parent families	3.01
% living in overcrowded households	2.88
% changed address within 1 year	2.68
% ethnic minorities	2.50

placed on them by these groups. For instance, the GPs surveyed considered that more work resulted from the 'elderly living alone group' than from the 'ethnic minorities group'. Talbot[3] and Smith[4] provide critiques of this index in the context of the NHS reforms.

The Townsend index

The Townsend index combines the scores on four census variables which are % unemployed, % overcrowded households, % households without a car and % households not owner-occupied. Each variable has equal weighting. Before variables are combined, they are transformed to a common scale.

National surveys

Often without going to the expense of conducting local surveys, useful information can be obtained from national surveys. Trends over time nationally are often reflected at the local level, and in the absence of local data extrapolation of national data to the local level can form the basis for planning.

The General Household Survey

The General Household Survey began in 1971. The sample frame is a carefully designed rotating representative sample of 15,000 private households (about 31,000 people) in the UK each year. In each selected household, all of the people aged 16 and over are interviewed. In addition, parents are questioned about the health and education of their children. The major topics covered at interview include housing, type of tenure and amenities. The questions on internal migration and employment cover past and potential migration, job satisfaction and reasons for absence. Educational qualifications are noted, as are schools attended. Some fertility data are noted, such as the number of children born into the present marriage and future expectations. In relation to health and health services, the occurrence of acute and chronic sickness, consultations with GPs, hospital visits and the use of other health and welfare services during the previous 2 weeks are recorded. Because the subjects are asked about any chronic or acute illnesses suffered in the 2 weeks prior to interview, estimates of the incidence of acute diseases and the prevalence of chronic disease can be made. However, the survey is not intended as a precise instrument for the surveillance of the incidence and prevalence of specific diseases, such as would meet the needs of those planning health services. Some topics are only covered sporadically. These include self-medication, smoking habits and time on hospital waiting lists.

The mechanics of the survey are that the sample is taken from the electoral register. It is a stratified clustered sample. Households in 60 local authorities are interviewed in any 1 year. In the following year, households in some of the same local authorities will be used plus new households in other local authorities. In the subsequent year, there will be a further reduction in the number of original local authorities used, so that in 5–6 years sample households from all local authorities will have been studied.

National Food Survey

Information about the changing food habits of the population can be obtained from the National Food Survey. It is based on food budgets of about 7500 households. The fieldwork takes place in 52 local authorities selected so as to be representative of the population at large. A proportion of local authorities are replaced for sampling purposes at the end of each calendar quarter. Examples of changes over time are shown in Table 4.3.

Table 4.3   Estimated food consumption (oz per person per week)

	1977	1987
Butter	4.70	2.14
Margarine	3.48	3.98
Eggs	4.00	2.89

Source: *Annual Abstracts of Statistics, 1989*. HMSO, London.

In general, dietary surveys are difficult to undertake and considerable expertise is required to conduct and interpret them. Self-completed food diaries are often not done satisfactorily and checklists of foods eaten while giving a qualitative view of diet often fail to yield good quantitative data.

Labour Force Survey

The Labour Force Survey is a voluntary and confidential survey carried out by OPCS on an annual basis. The first survey took place in 1973. The survey consists of two parts. There is a quarterly survey of about 15,000 households in the UK supplemented by a booster survey in the quarter March to May when approximately an additional 44,000 households are interviewed. The response ratio (see pp. 167–9) is about 85%. The population sampled is classified into economically active or inactive, and there is information on private household populations by ethnic group and economic activity. In addition, there are data on occupational mobility. The sampling has been designed so that extrapolation to the population of the UK is possible. It should be noted that the Labour Force Survey is currently the prime source of information on ethnicity.

Vital statistics

Vital statistics are 'measurements' of a community or population. They can tell us something about the size, age and health experience of the population. Census data, described above, are a component of the routine vital statistics information available in this country. Other components are explored below.

Births, marriages and deaths have been recorded for centuries; old parish registers contain them. However, these were not complete or compulsory. In London in the seventeenth century, Bills of Mortality were published, weekly broadsheets that listed for the London parishes the number of deaths and gave some indication of their cause. They tended to be purchased by the wealthier inhabitants of the city who would monitor plague deaths and quit the city if they foresaw an epidemic. In 1836, the Registrar's General Office was formed and this took over centrally the registration role for births, marriages and deaths, a role now performed by OPCS. In 1837, the registration of births, marriages and deaths by government enactment became compulsory in England and Wales. Under William Farr,[5] who has been described as the founder of medical statistics in this country, such data were used to describe the health of the country and what was happening to health over a period of time. The key to his work lay in relating population data to mortality data. This relationship was expressed as death rates.

Death rates

A rate can be calculated from the number of happenings in unit time divided by the population at risk. Thus the death rate for a population would be the number of deaths in the population in a year divided by the mid-year population at risk. This would express the overall death rate for that community, but the death rate could be broken down into age-specific death rates, e.g. infant mortality rates – these relate to deaths under 1 year.

Rates can be used to monitor the course of an epidemic. It would be helpful if the HIV/AIDS epidemic could be monitored by following death rates, but unfortunately it is difficult to collect accurate numerator and denominator data. The effect of interventions can be evaluated by clinical trials using case fatality rates as the end-point (see also Chapter 7).

Death certification

Although the coverage of death certification in the UK is good, i.e. almost a

100% of all deaths are reported, the quality of the information is not that high. There are two main parties concerned with providing information for the certificate: these are the *qualified informant* and a registered medical practitioner. The qualified informant is usually a close relative of the deceased, e.g. husband or wife. However, this does not always apply and the relationship can often be more tenuous. This can lead to misinformation, e.g. the wrong occupation of the deceased may be given. The doctor is responsible for completing parts 1 and 2 of the certificate: in part 1 should be listed the immediate cause of death plus conditions giving rise to it; and in part 2 should be listed other significant factors contributing to death but not the major factor. The subsidiary causes listed regrettably often depend on the whim of the doctor completing the certificate; some doctors go into greater detail than others. There is also a considerable body of evidence from comparison of the written death certificate with post-mortem findings that the clinical diagnosis can be in error. Persons using death rates for evaluative purposes should be aware of these problems.

Occupational mortality

Details of occupational mortality can be found in the Registrar-General decennial supplements. As already stated, errors can occur because the occupation of the deceased was not clearly known by the qualified informant or because the informant, particularly if a relative, overvalues the deceased's occupational status when the death certificate is completed. Other errors occur because occupation is often difficult to classify on the basis of the description given and because job changing can occur between census and death registration.

Occupational mortality is usually expressed through standardized mortality ratios (see below). Its computation requires knowledge of the size of the occupational group under consideration (from the census) and the number of deaths arising from the group (from death certificates).

The standardized mortality ratio (SMR)

Consider two populations: one has a death rate of 30 per 100,000 per year, the other has a death rate of 40 per 100,000 per year. On first thoughts, it would appear that the second population has worse health than the first. However, if on investigation it is noted that the second population has substantially more persons over the age of 65 years, then since the death rate is higher (by biological necessity) in the elderly, this fact could explain the higher death rate in the second population as compared to the first; thus our original first thoughts may be incorrect. This illustrates that when comparing populations, age structure needs to be taken into account. Another important variable is gender; for instance, on average, females have a longer life-span than males. To overcome these difficulties so that populations can be compared, a technique called 'standardization' is used. Standardization allows variations in age and sex structures among populations to be allowed for when considering mortality comparisons. Ward, district, regional or area mortality is compared with that of a standard population, usually the national population. The standardized mortality ratio (SMR) is defined as follows:

$$\text{SMR} = \frac{\text{Observed deaths}}{\text{Expected deaths}} \times 100$$

The observed deaths are the actual deaths in the population under study; the expected deaths are the deaths that would have been found if the population under study had the same risk of death in each age/sex group as the standard population. Details of how to calculate standardized mortality ratios are given in standard textbooks of epidemiology (see Further reading list). A high SMR (> 100) reflects poorer health than the standard (usually national), a low SMR (< 100) better than the standard; by definition, the SMR of the standard population is 100.

For instance, if for coronary heart disease a health authority had an SMR of 170 as compared to the SMR of 100 for England and Wales, the population of that health authority would be faring worse than the country as a whole in regard to that disease. This should alert the health authority to seek to find out the reasons. For example, on examination, it may be noted that their population smokes more than the national average. Cigarette smoking is a known risk factor for coronary heart disease. It may be that their health promotional programmes, unlike other parts of the country, are not producing beneficial behavioural changes.

There are some subtleties to the SMR which should be borne in mind. The SMR is particularly sensitive to differences in mortality between populations arising from fixed proportional change in mortality rates across the age bands, i.e. when the ratios of age-specific mortality rates between the study and reference populations are the same for each age band. Other patterns of mortality difference may not show up so strongly as differences in SMR. Moreover, when interesting differences in SMRs are found, it is then necessary to look – if feasible via age-specific mortality – at how in detail they arise. The choice of reference (standard) population is fairly arbitrary. It is sensible to use a reference population that obviously relates to or encompasses the particular populations being compared. Also, if secular trends in SMR among several places are being studied, the following factors should be considered:

1. Changes in mortality in each population as time progresses.
2. Changes in the mortality experiences of each population relative to the others as time progresses.

The former is best dealt with by choosing a reference population at the midpoint of the time interval being studied. For example, if trends in SMR are being examined for the period 1980–89, then the SMR should use England and Wales in 1984 or 1985 as the reference population. The latter issue is illuminated by using England and Wales reference populations for *each* of the years 1980–89.

The SMR is known technically as an indirect method of standardization. We have introduced it because it is the most commonly used in the health service. The alternative method, the direct method of standardization, gives an index which has the appearance of a death rate rather than, as is the case with the SMR, a ratio. The reader interested in pursuing this further is referred to epidemiological texts.

Morbidity indicators

Death rates are, apart from their intrinsic importance, useful proxies for the levels of ill-health (morbidity) in the population which arise from diseases with a fairly high case-fatality. Thus, if the case-fatality is 50%, it may *roughly* be assumed that at any time twice as many people are experiencing morbidity associated with the condition. However, many conditions which cause significant levels of morbidity and disability tend to have low case-fatalities. To take an extreme example, it would be absurd to use mortality rates for the common cold as a measure of the burden placed upon the community by this illness.

The two basic measures of morbidity are incidence and prevalence. The *incidence rate* is defined as the number of events that occur in a specified population in a specified period of time, e.g. the number of new cases of whooping cough reported in children 0–2 years old in 1 week. On the other hand, the *prevalence ratio* is the number of illnesses at any one time in specified population of known size, e.g. the number of children suffering from whooping cough per 1000 children aged 0–2 years on a specified day. In this case, on that specified day, both new cases and cases recovering from the disease would be included.

Incidence ratios are particularly useful for monitoring the course of an epidemic, whereas prevalence ratios are often important for service planning. A number of infectious diseases are notifiable, which include diphtheria, dysentery, encephalitis, food poisoning, infectious jaundice, measles, meningitis, mumps, pertussis (whooping cough), poliomyelitis, rubella (German measles), tetanus and other usually more rare diseases.

OPCS publishes statistics on infectious diseases. The system depends on the medical profession reporting such cases. Unfortunately, the level of reporting tends to vary. Doctors are more likely to report only what they consider serious conditions, and thus notification rates for poliomyelitis are likely to be better than those for measles. Nevertheless, changing patterns of reporting are helpful to those seeking to monitor epidemics.

Besides the legal requirement for the notification of certain infectious diseases, there are voluntary systems, e.g. notification of HIV infections and AIDS cases has been on a confidential voluntary basis. It is likely, however, that the notification rate considerably underestimates the true rate, and the same is true for other sensitive areas such as the usage of illegal drugs in the community; statistics available from the police are almost certainly a considerable underestimate. These reservations must be borne in mind when interpreting the data.

Apart from such inferences as can be drawn from mortality rates, incidence and prevalence measures do not routinely exist for most non-infectious diseases. The exceptions tend to be when population-based disease registers are created. For example, the national network of cancer registries provides valuable information on cancer registrations (proxy for incidence) and survival (duration of disease). If it is assumed that incidence and survival are constant, then disease prevalence may be estimated from the following relationship:

$$\text{Prevalence} = \text{incidence} \times \text{duration of disease}$$

Data from disease registries should not be taken at face value. Cancer registries differ considerably in the quality and timeliness of their data.

Given the paucity of routine information on morbidity and disability, it is often necessary to resort to *ad hoc* surveys.

Indicators of positive health

Morbidity indices measure ill-health, i.e. the lack of health or *negative health*. The converse of the negative health indicator is the positive health indicator. A positive health indicator measures things which promote and sustain health. These indicators are extremely hard to construct and use on a routine basis.

Two obtainable positive health indicators for the community are immunization uptake rates and cervical cytology screening rate. Breast screening rates will also be available in most districts during the 1990s.

Data sources relating to primary care

Surprisingly, routine data are relatively sparse, especially when one considers that the majority of contacts that the general public have with the health service are with general practice.

Family Health Service Authorities

Family Health Service Authorities (FHSAs) hold GP lists in their area. Unfortunately, these population lists are often in error, the error rates on addresses having been estimated to be as large as 25% (particularly in inner cities), but 10% is an often quoted figure. When patients move out of an area and transfer to another GP, there is a lag time before the patient record is removed from one FHSA and transferred to another. Patients also move house in an area without telling their GP or FHSA, so that although the same GP is retained the patient address is wrong. FHSAs are now moving to postcoding their GP lists. Many GPs have their own age/sex registers on computer. A spin off from the new GP contract, in consequence of the necessity for GPs to get good target rates for immunization and vaccination before payment, will be more accurate GP age/sex registers. The FHSAs will liaise with health authorities and share information so that in the future it will be easier to get a better picture of morbidity and mortality in a district or part of a district.

Practice process and outcome data

There is a network of GP practices which at selected times are prepared to keep a casebook of their workload over a short period. The results are then coded and these data form the basis for the Royal College of General Practitioners' national surveys. It is important to appreciate that participants in these surveys are enthusiastic volunteers. Their practices are not randomly distributed throughout the country, i.e. a non-representative sample is obtained. Nevertheless, provided the same practices are used, time-trend data can be obtained. Three national studies on morbidity in general practice have been published.[6,7] Also, a group of interested GPs act as sentinal practices for reporting infectious diseases, so allowing the Department of Health to monitor epidemics.

The recently introduced requirement that all general practices regularly health screen their patients aged over 75 years offers the prospect of a rich source of information about morbidity. However, to be worthwhile, the screening will have to be conducted to a common protocol and information will need to be recorded systematically.

General practitioners have started to produce annual reports for their FHSA. These should contain useful data on local morbidity. Initially, their content is likely to be variable but will become more consistent and useful if the FHSAs are able to persuade all practitioners in an area to report on the morbidity in their practice from, say, diabetes or angina.

Another approach is to link morbidity with prescribing data. General practitioners in the near future will receive better information on their use of drugs. It is possible to consider, for example, the usage of antidiabetic drugs as a proxy for diabetic morbidity in a practice. Similarly, for morbidity due to angina, a proxy could be the usage of nitrites.

The general practice research unit of the Royal College of General Practitioners has developed a diagnostic index which is condensed from the International Classification of Disease (ICD) codes and which the college considers suitable for GPs. Used in conjunction with the age/sex register of a practice, morbidity rates can be generated.

One GP, Dr Read, has developed a classification often referred to as the Read Code.[8] Copyright for this has been purchased by the NHS. It is likely to become the standard medical classification of medical terminology and medical practice in this country. It covers all major areas relating to practice from aetiology of disease through symptoms and signs to treatment of disease by medical and surgical means. It is a hierarchical system with five levels at present. Its text terms are associated with an alphanumeric code. In contrast to ICD9 and OPSC4, where there are at each level 10 options (the digits 0–9), the Read system uses upper- and lower-case letters and can produce 52 options. With the 5-digit code that is currently in use, there are over 600 million possible final items, so that the system has a lot of reserve capacity at present. Cross-referencing can occur with the ICD9 codes.

Data sources relating to hospitals

Following on from the recommendations of the Korner Committee,[9] a completely new routine data collection system was developed. This came into operation in 1987. Prior to that, the major source for process information was Hospital Activity Analysis (HAA). Data so obtained allowed length of stay, turnover interval and bed occupancy to be calculated. About 5% of patients seen by GPs are referred to hospital.

Hospital activity analysis

Until 1987, this was the major source for process information relating to the hospitals in the UK. It was based on information collected at the *end* of a stay in hospital; it covered every death and discharge from all hospitals. The data were regionally collated and a 1:10 sample, the Hospital Inpatient Enquiry (HIPE), was used nationally. There were separate systems for maternity and mental illness. Hospital admission data included demographic information on the patient and the type of admission. At discharge (or death), the data included date discharged, to where discharged (e.g. home, another ward, hospital, etc.), consultant seen and diagnosis. HAA data were used for planning and for evaluation. There were problems with the system, the three most important of which were:

1. The data that were produced were often grossly out of date; lag times of several years were quite common.
2. The system dealt with episodes and not patients, so that patient numbers per year were overestimated due to the difficulty of calculating readmission rates for patients. The overestimate was often of the order of 15%.
3. The data were often inaccurate and miscoding was relatively common.

In addition, patients in the maternity and psychiatric services were generally excluded. For these reasons, the system fell into disrepute.

Korner data sets

In 1979, a Royal Commission on the NHS stated: 'The information available to assist decision makers in the NHS leaves much to be desired.' The commission went on to say that the information produced was often late and of dubious accuracy. This led the Department of Health and Social Security (DHSS) to set up the Korner Committee with a remit to review existing health service information systems and to consider proposals for changes. Between 1982 and 1984, the Committee produced a number of reports dealing with information needs for particular purposes. Six main reports were produced: the first dealt with hospital facilities and diagnostic services, the second with patient transport, the third with manpower, the fourth with paramedical services, the fifth with community services and the sixth with finance.

The key concepts were that data collection should be linked with the districts and, associated with this, an identified minimum data set for specific parts of the health service. The steering group stated that they believed 'it is possible to identify a minimum set of data which should be used in all districts'. Moreover, they felt such data should be collected largely as a by-product of operational procedures.

The committee clearly went to considerable lengths to define a number of terms which had been loosely interpreted in the past and thereby introduce a national standard so that inter-district comparisons could take place. For example, a ward has to meet the following criteria: there must be a group of beds, there must be treatment facilities and it must be managed by a senior nurse.

Patient information systems

Computer systems are now in place in districts to collect within the hospital setting information on consultant episodes and ward stays. Information collection is initiated at the *beginning* of someone's stay in hospital. The consultant episode is the time a patient spends in the care of one consultant and the ward stay is the time a patient stays in one ward. The concept of the district spell was also developed, which is the total continuous stay of a patient in a hospital or hospitals in a particular district.

The first report of the Korner Committee recommended that the following information should be collected for patients admitted to hospitals: demographic details such as date of birth, sex, marital status and postcoded home address. Information should also be obtained on the method of admission (e.g. elective, emergency), the date of admission and a coded reference of the patient's usual GP. By specialities the code of every consultant responsible for care should be noted and the wards used should be coded. At the end of each consultant episode, the patient record should hold diagnostic information. This should be in ICD9 form (up to six diagnoses) and use OPCS operation codes. The patients should be classified (e.g. ordinary admission, day cases, etc.) and the date of their discharge noted. Deaths, if they occurred, should be registered.

For patients admitted to maternity wards it was recommended that there should be a minimum data set for the mother, a minimum data set for each baby, and each baby should have a delivery birth notification. There were special recommendations with regard to psychiatric hospitals. For instance, it was recommended:

> . . . that an annual census be carried out on an agreed day on all patients who have been in mental illness, mental handicap units or hospitals for a year or more, and on all detained patients.

It was also recommended that the use of electroconvulsive therapy be recorded.

The committee considered that data should be obtained on ward activity, but that the system of listing ward activity as 'activity as at midnight' be replaced by activity which had taken place in the previous 24 hours. Bed status (e.g.

Table 4.4 Out-patient non-attendance rates by speciality, North West Regional Health Authority 1988–89

General surgery	New out-patients			Reattendances			Total attendances		
	Attenders	DNA	%DNA	Attenders	DNA	%DNA	Attenders	DNA	%DNA
Lancaster	2 746	293	9.6	7 462	787	9.6	10 198	1 080	9.6
Blackpool	6 742	889	11.6	10 739	1 816	14.5	17 481	2 705	13.4
Preston	5 257	494	8.6	9 878	999	9.2	15 135	1 493	9.0
Blackburn	5 458	527	9.8	9 857	1 431	12.7	15 314	1 958	11.3
Burnley	4 536	524	10.4	10 203	1 639	13.8	14 739	2 163	12.8
West Lancashire	2 809	359	11.3	5 253	733	12.2	8 062	1 092	11.9
Chorley	3 705	274	6.9	4 592	426	8.5	8 297	700	7.8
Bolton	6 634	810	10.9	14 135	2 084	12.8	20 769	2 894	12.2
Bury	4 289	564	11.6	9 572	1 557	14.0	13 861	2 121	13.3
North Manchester	5 182	859	14.2	12 504	2 762	18.1	17 686	3 621	17.0
Central Manchester	4 781	984	17.1	15 826	4 051	20.4	20 607	5 035	19.6
South Manchester	9 353	1 266	11.9	19 746	3 450	14.9	29 099	4 716	13.9
Oldham	5 447	532	8.9	13 311	1 886	12.4	18 758	2 418	11.4
Rochdale	4 239	586	12.1	8 476	1 807	17.6	12 715	2 393	15.8
Salford	5 816	1 016	14.9	14 094	3 117	18.1	19 910	4 133	17.2
Stockport	5 358	576	9.7	9 541	1 495	13.5	14 899	2 071	12.2
Tameside	4 947	813	14.1	4 779	907	16.0	9 726	1 720	15.0
Trafford	4 123	589	12.5	8 522	1 648	16.2	12 645	2 237	15.0
Wigan	6 643	651	8.9	17 796	2 291	11.4	24 439	2 942	10.7
Speciality sub-total	98 065	12 606	11.4	206 275	34 886	14.5	304 340	47 492	13.5

Activity Data (Korner statistics).
Note variations in out-patient DNA (did not attend), e.g. between Chorley and Central Manchester.
Extreme figures, such as those noted for Central Manchester, merit further investigation by district management.

available, reserved, occupied, unoccupied) should be noted, and as well as noting patients who used a hospital bed the number of ward attenders (those patients not requiring a hospital bed) should also be recorded.

Recommendations were also made for a minimum data set for out-patients. Table 4.4 lists some activity data relating to out-patient non-attendance rates for surgery in the North Western Region in 1988–89.

The minimum data set covers district patient number, sex, date of birth, marital status, postcode of current home address, code of GP, category of patient, dates of appointment and source of initial attendance. This was categorized, e.g. self-referral, referral from A and E, following home visit by consultant, etc. The code of the consultant in charge and of the clinic was required as well as the date of discharge.

It was also recommended that activity data on operating theatre usage (e.g. scheduled sessions held, scheduled sessions cancelled, cases outside scheduled sessions) should be gathered, as well as activity data relating to day care and the diagnostic services, e.g. tests requested. In the 1980s, the NHS invested considerable resources in patient administration systems that could handle Korner data.

Community services

In the introduction to the fifth Korner Report, the following statement is made:

> In structuring information about community health services we have drawn an important distinction between:
> (a) services to the community;
> (b) services in the community.

Examples of services to the community are immunization, health surveillance and the early detection of disease. Within this area would fall contact tracing, cervical cancer and breast cancer screening, and health promotion and education. The report recommended that for each programme data should be assembled annually which gave target level of coverage, estimated target population, projected expenditure, level of service provided and the coverage which had been achieved as compared to target.

For care in the community, information about patient care services should be classified under three headings: general services (i.e. district nursing), mental illness services (i.e. community psychiatric nursing) and others. For each area, an annual programme should be assembled which should include a statement of local policy and objectives, information about related services (local authority, voluntary), estimated present and future catchment populations, projected expenditure, estimated actual expenditure and patient activity. The data on client activity should note whether initial contact was made or not, location of contact, the source of referral for all initial contacts and, for all initial contacts and first contacts in the financial year, the client's age (in eight age bands) and sex.

The NHS information system which has developed out of the Korner reports allows for a much better analysis of process information than was possible with HAA. It will also enable activity to be linked with resources more effectively and for more reliable costing of procedures to be made. The identification and use of diagnostic-related groups (see below) will enhance this. The system will also produce some outcome data which will be more reliable than in the past.

The contracting process within the NHS which commenced in April 1991 means that both the purchaser and the provider will require accurate and timely information on process and outcome so that bills can be paid and provider performance monitored. The new providers – the NHS Trusts – will need to produce such information.

Diagnostic-related groups

Diagnostic-related groups (DRGs)[10] is a classification initially developed at Yale University for classifying case types and linking these with resources. They enabled a prospective payment system to be developed with the objective of controlling charges more strictly. DRGs describe the type of patient discharged from acute care hospitals.

Patients are classified into about 500 classes, each defined by one or more of the following variables: principal diagnosis, surgical procedures, additional diagnoses (co-morbidities and complications), age, sex and discharge disposition. Within each group, the resources utilized are expected to be similar, i.e. the groups were designed to be clinically coherent in that they resulted in a set of clinical responses which led to similar overall costs. The profile of services ordered by the clinician is expected to be similar for all patients treated in a given DRG, and though in practice one patient may cost more and another may cost less than the DRG cost, the DRG cost is expected to be a sensible average cost for providing the service for such patients.

The use by the NHS of DRGs has considerable implications for managers and doctors. It invokes product line management into the health service. The product is the patient, the product manager the clinician who is responsible for putting together a package of services (outputs) that are necessary for the patient's care. For example, a patient needing a cholecystectomy would require while in hospital so many hours of surgical time, so many days of hotel costs, so many laboratory tests, etc. Each element could be costed (see Table 4.5) so that the expected cost of treatment could be forecast. Budgets would be aggregations of a hospital's mix of cases in terms of components of each case type and their cost.

The actual costs incurred could be compared with expected cost to see the source of any variation. While the clinicians are product managers, the departmental heads would be responsible for managing the conversion of inputs (staff time, materials, equipment) to outputs (hours of nursing or paramedical care, X-rays, laboratory tests, etc.) as efficiently as possible. Part of the *resource management initiative*[11] is to prepare clinicians for the role of product manager (see p. 53). The concept of product line management is linked to the Donabedian analysis of the health service having three components, i.e. structure, process and outcome (see Chapter 1). In product line management, the structure lets the clinician take the role of product manager and the process is the packages of services. In both, the patient is the treated object.

Criteria for evaluating case-mix classification

Hornbrook[12] suggested the following criteria:
1. *Reliability*: the methodology should not be susceptible to random errors and consistent answers should be obtained when raw data are processed.
2. *Validity* on three dimensions: content validity (in that it is representative and comprehensive), predictive validity (in that there is an ability to predict some future outcome) and construct validity (in that one can explain differences in a theoretically coherent way).
3. *Sensitivity*: the measures should enable discrimination to occur between hospitals. Nowadays, discrimination between consultants working in the same field is required.

Table 4.5   Skeleton of a costing table for DRGs

	LAB COSTS	XRAY COSTS	PHYSIO COSTS	PSYCHOL COSTS	ETC	NURSING COSTS	OP ROOM COSTS	ANAESTHETIC COSTS	ETC	TOTAL
DRG										
DRG										

PHYSIO, physiotherapy; PSYCHOL, psychology; OP ROOM, operation room = theatre.

4. *Cost-effectiveness*: the 'least cost method' should be used so long as performance is not affected, i.e. if two treatments produce the same outcome, the least cost method should be chosen.
5. *Flexibility*: the methodology should be capable of being used for a variety of purposes.
6. *Acceptability*: the methodology should be acceptable to all users.

It is possible to challenge DRGs on the grounds that they do not fully meet these criteria. For instance, acceptability and cost-effectiveness are two areas where they are susceptible to questioning. However, they do enable some feel for case-mix to become part of the routine information system of hospitals.

Isoresource groups

DRGs are isoresource groups. This is a confusing term, since these groups are not defined on costs of expected resource use (e.g. patients classified as £1000 per case patients or £2000 per case patients) but on the ability to discriminate between costs of treatment. DRGs have been criticized in that they fail to take into account the more seriously ill patients. Co-morbidity (i.e. illnesses associated with the main disease) weighting is an attempt to meet this criticism, though it can be stated that co-morbidities cover a wide range of illness of differing severity.

Obtaining a DRG

Medical staff are required to state the diagnosis and any surgical action taken if applicable. The ICD9 and OPCS4 surgical codes need to be converted into ICD-9-CM (clinical modification) codes. The NHS has produced a computer software program called the Grouper Program which can assign in-patients to DRGs. This program is suitable for records coded in ICD-9-CM. Major Diagnostic Categories (MDCs) are 23 broad categories of disease into which DRGs are grouped, e.g. diseases of the nervous system, circulatory system and digestive system. These are stratified by medical or surgical procedures, by age and by co-morbidities or complications to arrive at the correct DRG.

The Grouper program

The Grouper program first checks the data fed in for any incompatibilities, e.g. if sex is given as male some error must have occurred if the operation is one on the uterus. It then follows a series of decision pathways to arrive at the unique DRG. These can be represented as a 'tree'. Decision trees have been constructed for each of the 23 MDCs (see Fig. 4.3). On average, each MDC has about 20 DRGs in it. However, there is quite a wide range. Figure 4.4 displays the information needed for obtaining a DRG for a particular case. The example deals with the following case history:

A female aged 80 years had colicky abdominal pain for approximately 3 days. The patient had been nauseated and had vomited three times in the

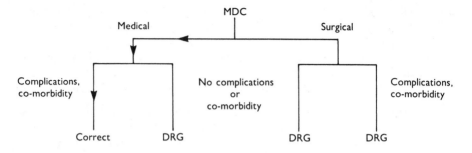

Fig. 4.3   A decision tree for major diagnostic category. If for this MDC one is dealing with medical conditions, the arrowed path is followed to arrive at the correct DRG.

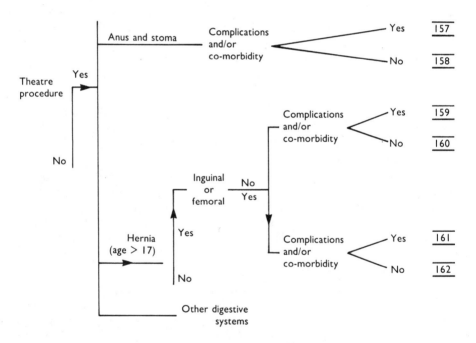

Decision path: Yes theatre procedure, Yes hernia,
Yes age > 17, Yes inguinal or femoral,
Yes complications and/or co-morbidities

Based on DRG's 5th Revision. Definition Manual Health System International 1988

Fig. 4.4   The information required to calculate a particular DRG: Diseases and disorders of the digestive system (MDC6). The correct DRG is DRG161.

past 24 hours. She also suffered from shortness of breath. On examination, there was a tender irreducible lump in the left groin. A raised jugular pulse was seen and there was pitting ankle oedema. The patient was diagnosed as having an obstructed femoral hernia and also congestive cardiac failure. The diagnosis of obstructive femoral hernia was confirmed on operation. An emergency repair of femoral hernia with sutures was carried out. Post-operatively, the patient developed a urinary tract infection which responded to treatment. The patient was discharged after 8 days.

The case was coded as follows:

Final diagnosis	*ICD9 codes*
● Primary:	
Obstructed femoral hernia	552.2
● Secondary:	
Congestive cardiac failure	428.0
Urinary tract infection	041.4
Procedure	*OPCS4 code*
Repair of femoral hernia with sutures	T 22.3
– – – – → MCD 6	
– – – – → DRG 161	

Outliers

DRGs can be used for evaluation when length of stay is at issue. *Outliers* are extreme cases within a given DRG. They can be defined as those patients with lengths of stay greater than two standard deviations above the mean length of stay of all similar patients. Such outliers usually need to be investigated. Often, an investigation will reveal that they have been miscoded, but if this is not the case then other reasons need to be identified. Persons using DRGs should be aware that trimmed data (Fig. 4.5) are often used to calculate the mean length of stay. Trimmed data are data from which the outliers have been removed; unless one can be certain that outliers represent miscoding and that miscoding applies equally to all diagnoses within a DRG, trimming is a statistically invalid technique which may lead to serious bias.

Two problems that have occurred with the use of DRGs are 'DRG creep', the ability to shift a patient to a higher paying DRG category with minor changes in coding, and the inability for DRGs to account adequately for severity of illness. The use of co-morbidities and/or complications without severity ratings lead to the same DRG and is an indication of the insensitivity of the method.

Audit

Audit is a method of evaluation that has become more common in the NHS following the Government White Paper on the reorganization of the NHS and

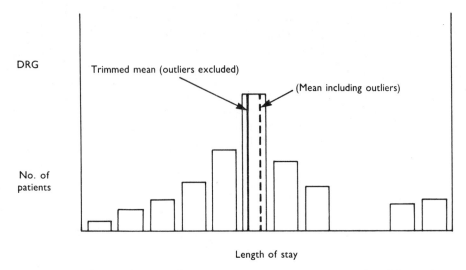

Fig. 4.5 Outliers and trimmed means. Sometimes upon examination, false outliers occur due to miscoding or clerical errors – outliers should be checked. Outlier defined as + 2S.D. from the mean.

the setting up of district audit committees. These are committees set up by districts to collect data systematically on audit and to see that appropriate management action is taken following on from the results of audits received. Medical audit has become prominent and received special funding, but it should be borne in mind that audit is becoming well-developed within nursing practice and is likely to be taken on by other paramedical disciplines. It is important to be clear about the terms used in the audit area, otherwise this can lead to confusion. Some common terms are defined below.

Medical audit

Definition: the following definition is given in NHS paper No. 6:

> Medical Audit can be defined as the systematic critical analysis of the quality of medical care, including the procedures used for diagnosis and treatment, the use of resources and the resulting outcome and quality of life for the patient.

Purpose: the White Paper states:

> An effective programme of audit will help to provide the necessary assurance to doctors, patients and managers that the best quality of service is being achieved within the resources available.

Possible benefit of audit:

1. Improves patient outcome.
2. Improves patient quality of life.

3. Educative function for junior staff training.
4. Results in more cost-effective use of resources.

Possible disadvantages of audit:

1. A critical analysis of the quality of medical care takes professional time. There is a reciprocal relationship between quality of service and quantity of service and managers must accept in the first instance that a major audit initiative in a hospital can result in a reduction in the quantity of service.
2. Computer costs can be considerable both for capital equipment and for equipment maintenance and licensing agreements.
3. There will be infrastructure support costs, e.g. for medical audit assistants or for computer personnel.

Levels of audit: the following levels could be considered:

1. At the individual consultant level, a consultant systematically reviews the work of his unit with junior staff.
2. Peer review audit is where members of a discipline review each other's work. For instance, a group of psychiatrists may meet and review the outcome of a specific form of behavioural therapy on their patients. This approach can be extended to interdisciplinary peer reviews, e.g. anaesthetists and surgeons may review peri-operative deaths.
3. External audits have often been initiated by the Royal Colleges. An example is the confidential enquiry into peri-operative mortality. External audits could be carried out at the national, regional or district levels.

Types of audit:

1. *Effectiveness*: under this heading outcomes can be considered, e.g. death audits see if any deaths are preventable. Quality of life audits would also fall under this heading.
2. *Efficiency*: consideration of the most effective use of resources to produce the desired outcome, e.g. was there unnecessary utilization of supportive services?
3. *Equity*: audits in this area are designed to determine if there are any geographical, social or ethnic barriers to uptake of services.
4. *Relevance to need*: audits in this area are designed to answer the following question: does the pattern of medical activity actually relate to the needs of the population?

Clinical audit

Clinical audit is a systematic and critical analysis of the quality of professional care. The term 'clinical audit' includes medical audit but covers audit by other professionals either alone or in conjunction with doctors (e.g. nursing audit, physiotherapy audit).

Resource management initiative

The resource management initiative is the name given to the NHS Management Board project for developing improved arrangements for managing resources in health authorities. In essence, it is an information technology initiative to enable the identification of costs generated by individual clinicians. Clinicians receive the information generated and this feedback could lead to a modification of practice. Such cost identification is important when conducting efficiency audits, e.g. comparative costs of two types of treatment with the same outcome. Another component of the resource management initiative is to increase the managerial skills of clinicians.

Quality assurance

The quality assurance process is a clinical and managerial framework that ensures a systematic and continuous monitoring and evaluation of agreed levels of service and care provision. Many districts now employ a quality assurance officer who works with a quality assurance committee to define and monitor standards of service. Action can be taken following from the results of the audits received.

Medical and clinical audit (outlined above) may be viewed as part of overall quality initiatives. Figure 4.6 summarizes how work on audit could be classified on a three-dimensional matrix and Fig. 4.7 gives an example of a form which could be used by an audit committee.

Performance indicators

All services need to be evaluated and the DHSS (now the Department of Health) developed performance indicators (PIs) with that in view. PIs are intended to be practical and useful tools for management. The approach adopted was to derive a number of crude indicators of performance from routine data sources so that comparisons (e.g. inter-district or inter-speciality) could be made. The devisers

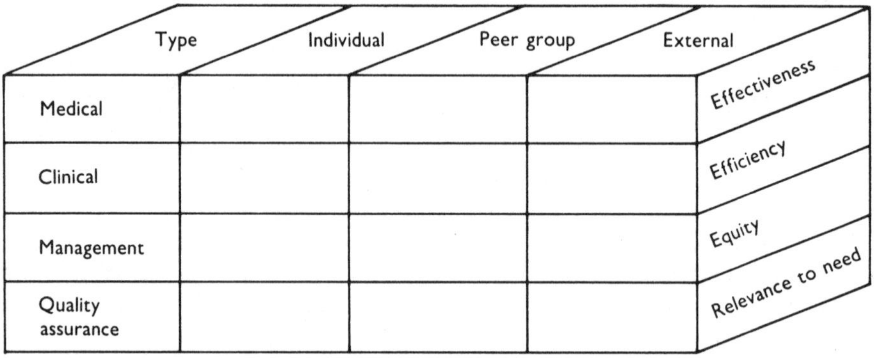

Fig. 4.6 Classification of audit along three different axes.

Form of audit		Type		Level	
Medical audit	☐	Effectiveness	☐	Individual firm	☐
Clinical audit	☐	Cost-efficiency	☐	Single discipline peer review	☐
Other	☐	Medical management	☐	Interdisciplinary peer review	☐
				External	☐

Period of audit ....

Topic audited (not more than 50 words) ....

....

....

....

Major finding 1. ....

2. ....

3. ....

4. ....

5. ....

Action resulting ....

....

....

....

....

Does management need to be informed?   ☐ Yes   ☐ No

If yes, what action is required ....

....

....

Are there any resource implications?   ☐ Yes   ☐ No

If yes, specify ....

....

....

Date management informed ....

Management response ....

Date returned from management ....

Fig. 4.7 Specimen audit report form.

of the present PIs realized that an analysis of information can only be as good as the data which is fed into it (i.e. if garbage goes in garbage comes out) and recognized that inaccuracies occurred. However, they considered that inaccuracies were not sufficient to prevent implementation of the system. PIs are indicators and not measures of performance. They provide pointers to areas which merit further consideration and investigation. Average PIs should not be used as 'standards' or 'norms'. More than 500 PIs have been developed for health service use.

In general, they are ratios – there is a numerator and a denominator. They can roughly be divided into three groups: clinical PIs, manpower PIs and financial PIs. An example of a manpower PI is the number of health visitors per 100,000 population. An example of a financial PI is the cost of a bed in geriatrics per day.

Clinical Performance Indicators

Clinical PIs are mainly concerned with some features of *process*, consistent with the product line concept as mentioned with DRGs. Length of stay, turnover interval and bed occupancy are three common clinical PIs. If a patient were to occupy a bed on a ward for 9 days, a second patient that same bed for 10 days and a third patient for 11 days, then the average length of stay for the three patients is 10 days (see Fig. 4.8). If this average length of stay held throughout the year and one assumes that ward was not functioning for 5 days per year, then 36 people could be processed through that bed. However, there is a delay between one person vacating the bed and another being admitted to it, i.e. the 'turnover interval'. If one assumes that this is 2 days, then only 30 persons (360/12) could possibly be processed through the bed. This would be the maximum bed occupancy. If in fact only 24 people occupied the bed in the year, then the percentage bed occupancy would be 80%. Table 4.6 shows the length of stay, turnover interval and throughput for two specialities in a district in the North Western Region; these findings prompted an investigation of these specialities.

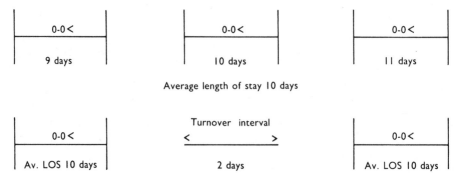

Fig. 4.8 Illustration of the relationship between average length of stay, turnover interval and bed occupancy.

Table 4.6 Illustration of use of performance indicators

Performance indicators	Speciality	
	Paediatrics	*Ophthalmology*
Length of stay	H	L
Turnover interval	H –	L –
Throughput	L	H

An 'L' means that the district ranking was in the lower extreme range and a 'H' that it was in the higher exteme range. A L – or H – indicates district ranking was not in extreme lower or upper range but in next lowest or highest range.

An example of performance indicators for two specialities in a North Western Region district. These alerted the district to investigate further. Further investigation allowed paediatric beds to be reduced and throughput to be increased, and for provision to be made for day case cataract surgery and medical manpower increases. Low length of stay and very high throughput can be a sign of considerable pressure on staff.

Following up PIs can generate a lot of work and it is important that managers don't come to hasty, ill-informed conclusions. Consider two surgeons, one in district A whose patients have an average length of stay of 15 days, and a second in district B whose patients have an average length of stay of 10 days. It cannot immediately be concluded that the surgeon in district A is inefficient. There are many reasons that could account for the difference, e.g. differences in case-mix, the inability of one surgeon to discharge his or her cases because of inadequate support from social services, the inability of one surgeon to get access to operating theatre time, the cancellations of operating lists because of a shortage of anaesthetists and differences in post-operative infection rates. This is not meant to be a comprehensive list of the possible causes of the differences between the two surgeons as regards the average length of stay of their patients, and, as can be appreciated, to disentangle these threads would require a great deal of effort. The difficult management decision is when and when not to embark on this level of effort.

Sources of data

Table 4.7 lists sources of some of the information mentioned in this chapter. Appendix A goes into more detail about how to obtain information. The reader should not forget that most DHAs and FHSAs have information officers who can be very helpful in these matters. Moreover, medical librarians, whether at local hospital libraries or university libraries, are familiar with diverse sources of information whether documented on paper, microfiche, CD-ROM disk or large computer databases.

Table 4.7   Some routine sources of data

Areas of interest	Source
Demographic data	
Estimated present population	OPCS population estimates
5-year population projection by age bands	OPCS population projections
Ethnic information	Census, Labour Force Survey
Deprivation, Jarman 8	*British Medical Journal*, **289**, 1587–92 (1984)
Housing	National Dwelling Survey
Activity data	
Process Data Hospital	Korner data KO forms, RHAs in England. (KARS) KES data, RHAs
Process Data Community	Korner data KC KT forms, RHAs in England
Hospitalization rates	Department of Health PIs, the regions
Performance indicators	Department of Health
Health and disease data	
Data relating to births	OPCS VS1 Monitor
Perinatal mortality rates	OPCS VS1 Monitor
Infant mortality rates	OPCS VS1 Monitor
Abortions	OPCS Monitor AB
Deaths by selected causes	OPCS Monitor VS3
SMR selected causes of death	Regions
Infectious diseases	OPCS Monitors MB, WR
Morbidity	General Household Survey, Royal College of General Practitioners

Chapter 5

Some basic economic concepts and their uses

Introduction

It is daunting to be told that in order to conduct worthwhile evaluations of service effectiveness and to use the findings of such evaluations in an informed way, it is necessary to understand economics. Nevertheless, this is true. It is a challenge which cannot be shirked.

We are not economists, but through our service and academic work we have come to appreciate the added dimension that economic thought adds to evaluation and we have been fortunate in having access to health economists with whom to collaborate. The reader is no more expected to become an economist than we are. However, the economist is as vital to an evaluation team as the statistician. Collaboration cannot be effective unless there is a shared understanding of some basic concepts of this science of scarcity. Moreover, an appreciation of economic ideas is essential to an understanding of the opportunities and challenges arising for health service planning and decision making from the reforms to the NHS (these are discussed in Chapter 12).

The next section introduces some fundamental concepts, and their importance should, for the moment, be taken on trust. It is followed by sections which show how these ideas are applied in the health service and their relevance should become apparent.

Basic concepts

Underlying the use of the terms we shall introduce is the key relationship between 'consumers' and 'producers'.

The consumer

Consumers are largely interested in *utility*, i.e. the satisfaction derived from any particular product. Much of the time we are trading off one utility against

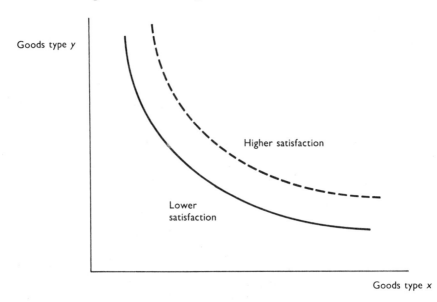

Fig. 5.1   An indifference curve. At any point on the curve, the customer is neither worse nor better off, he or she is indifferent. There are, however, different satisfaction levels. Within those, goods type *y* and goods type *x* can substitute for each other.

another (we can have our cake and eat it) and the balance between different utilities can be calculated in the form of an indifference curve for each individual (Fig. 5.1). Indifference curves:

- are negative, indicating that customers prefer more to less goods;
- are convex to the origin, in order to comply with the laws of diminishing marginal rate of substitution; and
- never cross each other.

Generally, the height of the curve indicates a level of satisfaction, because the customer has more goods.

The situation is complicated because products are usually neither homogeneous nor identical. They can all be regarded as consisting of 'bundles of attributes', and each attribute may, for example, relate to the status of the product, or to the process of acquisition, or to aesthetic or purely psychological considerations. In this context, a 'product' can be a tangible artefact, or an invisible but highly important service.

The relationship between the price which has to be paid for each product and the quantity which a consumer is prepared to purchase, is the *demand curve*; generally, it has a negative slope (i.e. as price goes up demand goes down), but this is not always so. In calculating such a curve, we look at the impact of, say, unit change in price compared with unit change in quantity

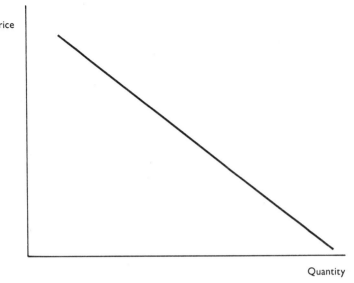

Fig. 5.2   A demand curve. The slope is nearly always negative.

purchased. This unit change is referred to as *marginal*. This is an essential economic concept since most of our decisions effect changes at the margin of what we are doing, rather than the total experience hitherto.

The relationship between price and quantity is measured as *elasticity*. The slope of the demand curve in Fig. 5.2 is negative because:

1. A positive *substitution effect* operates. As the price of a commodity declines, customers will try to increase their satisfaction by substituting their cheaper commodity for another; whole price has not declined.
2. An income effect tends to reinforce the substitution effect, i.e. customers tend to buy more when they have higher income levels.

Demand tends to be more *elastic* at higher prices. It can be seen from Fig. 5.3 that a price reduction at the top of the price range has a greater effect on the quantity demanded than a similar price reduction at lower levels.

All this assumes that a consumer is aware of the price of a product, and is quite clear about the utility. However, in real life, this is often far from true; there is always an element of *risk* – the element of uncertainty which we may attempt to cope with by calculating probabilities (the betting odds for or against a certain event).

The *opportunity cost* is usually all too clear; if I purchase one item I have to forgo another.

The producer

Any good, whether it is a tangible product or an intangible service, requires *factors of production*. These generally comprise *capital* (e.g. equipment) and

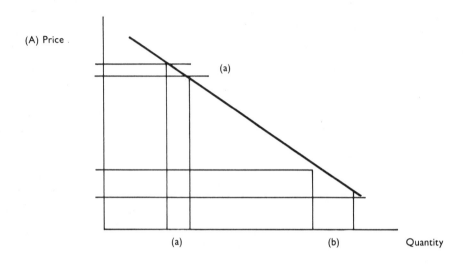

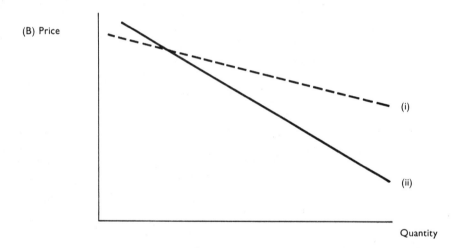

Fig. 5.3   Elasticity. (A). From the demand curve, it can be seen that change at a higher price level (a) has more effect than change at a lower level (b). (B) The slope of the line indicates the elasticity: (i) is more elastic than (ii), i.e. a given change in price has a greater effect on the quantity purchased.

labour. The quantity of goods which can be produced can be varied by altering either the capital or labour. The resulting output will depend on the relationship between capital and labour, and also on the mixture of goods being produced. Continuing to increase one factor of production (e.g. more equipment) may not necessarily result in similar increases in output (if more skilled manpower is needed); this can be demonstrated as *diminishing returns* (more accurately

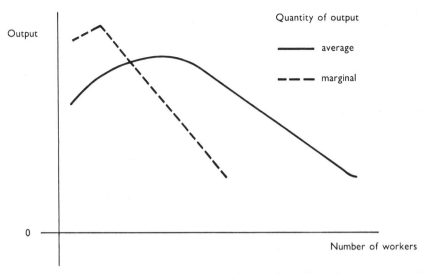

Fig. 5.4 Diminishing marginal returns. As the number of workers increases, the average output increases initially and then falls; as the number of workers increases, the marginal output rises briefly and then drops markedly.

diminishing marginal returns). This is illustrated in Fig. 5.4. This is not an economic theorem, it is a simple statement concerning physical relations that have been observed in a real economic world.

As the number of workers increases, the average output per worker rises initially and then falls. The marginal output (i.e. that additional output secured by increasing the labour force) rises briefly and then falls.

The costs of production may be *fixed* (relatively unchanging over time, as in equipment, buildings, vehicles) or *variable* (liable to alter with quantity of goods produced, as with part-time labour or consumables). The cost of manufacturing one more product or service is known as the *marginal cost*. Producers examining their costs may take the overall total and average this by unit of output in the long run, or they may prefer to look at the average variable costs, or they may see how marginal costs change over time and with different outputs. This is illustrated in Fig. 5.5.

The price paid for each product results in *revenue*; the additional revenue for every additional unit of output is the *marginal revenue*. In the long run, maximum profit is always earned when the output is set at the point where the marginal cost equals the marginal revenue, which in turn is set by a price set at the corresponding position on the demand curve.

Fixed costs remain steady: they are incurred when nothing is produced as well as when there is high output. Variable costs change with the quantity produced.

In the same way that consumers have a demand curve, producers have a *supply curve*; they will, however, wish to produce more output as price increases, so the curve is generally positive (see Fig. 5.6).

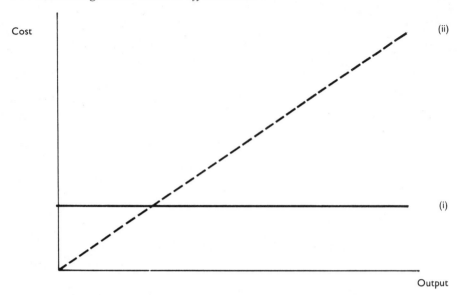

Fig. 5.5 Fixed and variable costs. (i) *Fixed costs*: the level stays the same whether there is zero output or a lot of output; (ii) *variable costs*: the level rises in relation to the level of output.

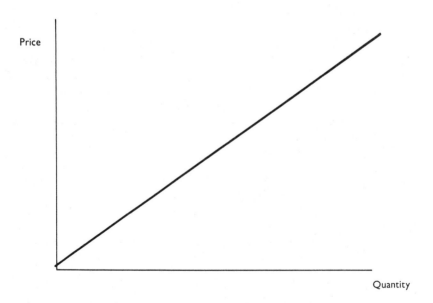

Fig. 5.6 A supply curve. The slope is virtually always positive.

Consumers and producers

The producer wants to maximize profits and the consumer wants to maximize utility. Profits depend on costs and the revenue generated by varying quantities of sales. Utility will be perceived in terms of income, the quantity of goods available and competition. The price–quality relationship is central. This is a complicated area of economics, partly because the theory of pricing is actually far from simple, and also because the understanding of perceived quality is difficult. For example, research has shown that the price of computers relates to many attributes, including their speed of operation, their capacity, their physical size and also to time – computers are generally getting cheaper.

Competition is about consumers and producers negotiating together in the same market. In crude terms, there are three types of competition: 'perfect' competition, monopoly and oligopoly. *Perfect competition* applies to the 'efficient' situation where there are lots of very similar small producers who are able to enter or leave the market with ease, where consumers and producers are all equally well informed, and where (above a certain level of production) maximim profit is made when the marginal cost of production equals the market price (revenue).

In a *monopoly*, there is only one producer who is expected to charge more and produce less than a competitive industry, and to price discriminately (e.g. off-peak travel or electricity) to keep output at a competitive level. A situation where there is a single purchaser is a *monopsony*.

In an *oligopoly*, there are only a few firms competing and they tend to have very similar prices. This seems to happen not necessarily through overt collusion but through price leadership (i.e. one firm sets the tone for the others), rules which are common to the whole industry, and through agreed focal points for prices. Identical pricing tends to be inhibited by decisions on the right price ('what happens if we go a little cheaper?'), allocating market shares, detecting cheating, communicating in a hostile environment, reacting to changes in demand or cost conditions (each firm will differ) and setting up entry barriers (this is not an easy field to get into).

It is generally assumed that there is some sort of finite market for a product and producers compete for a share of that market. *Market share* depends on buyer power, barriers to entry (can we afford to go in?), barriers to exit (can we afford to get out?) and a number of other factors.

The final concept to be mentioned relates to time. Decisions are not always based in the here and now, they often involve the future. To deal with this, economists have developed the process of *discounting*. A pound spent today is worth more than a pound which we might spend tomorrow. An asset worth a pound today will also be worth less tomorrow, independent of any depreciation. This is regardless of any inflation effect.

The special contribution of health economics

The foregoing is an attempt to give, briefly, a taste of some of the concepts which the science of economics covers. Each concept is in fact extremely complicated and would justify several books on its own. Health economists have special expertise in applying these concepts to our experiences of life and death, health and ill-health, and all the complicated notions which contribute to our ideas of the quality of life. They link these values with their financial implications, both for the provider institutions and for the individual consumers, and understand the strengths and weaknesses of the financial data available in the health service and elsewhere for these calculations.

Using economic concepts in the NHS

Economics is the science of scarcity. But how relevant is all this to evaluation and to the NHS? For a start, despite government spending exceeding £23 billion annually, health service demands exceed supply: there is scarcity. So economic concepts are highly relevant.

We make assumptions about utility and a consumer's (patient's) indifference curve. For example, it seems to be agreed that, for elective surgery, patients would prefer a short waiting time to geographical convenience if there has to be a trade-off between them. In the past, we have sometimes tended to think that it is reasonable to trade-off a surgeon's technical competence against his or her competence in personal relationships; fortunately, the view that one excludes the other is decreasingly tenable.

For providing units, marginal changes in activity will relate to marginal changes in cost – and the necessity to reconsider a price will depend on the form of service agreement already negotiated. There will also be quality enhancements to a service and these too should be regarded as essential components in the calculation relating to price and quality. A change in quality as well as a change in output quantity may have tremendous implications for the marginal change in cost or price.

We probably do not have enough experience yet to understand the price elasticity of various health services, but we do need to be aware of the price elasticity of a number of goods that affect health. For example, within a limited range, cigarettes tend to be price elastic, and therefore the Royal Colleges have begged the Chancellor to increase tobacco tax and cigarette prices to try and reduce their consumption. The health promotion strategy of making healthy choices easy choices relates to price elasticity, e.g. wholemeal *vs* white bread, polyunsaturated and mono-unsaturated fats. Admission rates in terms of hospital use may be elastic to bed availability and distance from hospital, rather than simple clinical need.

Communicating the risk involved in accepting a service is still far from straightforward. For some procedures, the probability of an adverse outcome can be quantified, as with, for example, amniocentesis to detect chromosomal abnormalities, where there is a definite associated risk that normal pregnancies (about 1 in 200) will abort. With new drugs and new treatments the risk is unquantified because there is no experience and no information.

Within the hospital, wards and nurses are factors of production. They generally represent the fixed cost. The number of drugs, bandages and investigations will vary with the number of patients; these will be variable costs. A very high proportion of hospital costs are fixed; that leaves very little room for flexibility in effecting cost reductions, if it is only the variable costs which are amenable to change. The marginal cost of, say, admitting one more patient will also vary. If the ward is already staffed and has a number of empty beds, the marginal cost will be minimal; if the ward is full, but the admission is still required and a whole new ward has to be opened up as a result, the marginal cost will be huge.

If a hospital can only afford to employ a certain number of nurses, there will have to be decisions about where to deploy them. Keeping a general medical ward open may mean, for example, that intensive care beds have to close. The opportunity costs of the alternatives may have to be measured in terms of intangibles, such as the impact on the quality of care available to patients or the effect on staff morale, as well as the financial implications of the reluctance of purchasers to refer patients to a hospital which lacks either a general medical ward, or where a number of intensive care beds have had to close.

We make tremendous assumptions about the utility of providing health services in the first place. We have no instruments for measuring or proving many of these assumptions. Presumably, patients do benefit from contact with health visitors, from having their hernias repaired, from coming into hospital with a stroke. But we are at an extremely early and very crude stage in attempting to unravel the bundle of attributes associated with each intervention. We seem to believe that consumers are only fit to comment on what professionals may perceive as relatively trivial attributes: the hotel services, such as heating, lighting and quality of food. We do not explore the competence with which service providers attempt to communicate the intention of their intervention, let alone monitor whether or not they achieve it.

We have a great deal of thinking still to do about competition. There are undoubtedly market segments at which producers should target services, e.g. the elderly, the young married and children. We remain unclear about whether or not we would wish to approach a situation which could be described as a perfect market, or if we are content with oligopoly, or in many places where there is only one hospital, a monopoly.

Applying economic concepts to service evaluation

Cost–benefit

Cost–benefit studies are probably the most frequent type of evaluation to which managers will be exposed. Their interpretation can also be the most difficult, since they can be used to present, vehemently, one side of an argument, while simulating objectivity. At their simplest, they present a summary of the costs which are incurred in order to achieve a given benefit. We have already hinted at some of the complexities of defining 'costs'; benefits, in terms of derived utility, are also vulnerable to being dealt with far too superficially.

The *costs* which are used in any evaluation can be judged in terms of their breadth, relevance, accuracy, type (fixed/variable) and interrelationships (opportunity, marginal, time-scale).

The breadth of costs means the extent to which allowance is made for the extent to which people are affected by a health service decision. For example, it would be possible to argue that doctors should only provide out-patient services in one location because that would save the NHS the costs of their travel to several locations. The argument focuses very narrowly on one cost only; it ignores the cost to patients, who may have to pay their own travel expenses and who may lose pay because so much time has to be taken off work in order to get to hospital. Health economists are particularly skilled at identifying the range of social costs which may be incurred by an apparent 'cost-saving' decision in the NHS.

It is thus tempting to list all possible costs which could be incurred by everyone, in order to seem to be fair and just. However, not all costs are relevant. For example, costs of low pay are immaterial in discussing the time required to transport very elderly people to a service such as a day hospital. Other costs, or disbenefits, will be far more important, such as loss of dignity, or so much time taken travelling that there is little left to use or enjoy the service provided.

Costs are an attempt to express in similar financial terms what has to be paid for something to be obtained. As such, they have the tremendous advantage of expressing all 'payments' in similar, and thus comparable, currency. They can, however, be extremely difficult to assess accurately. For example, what are the costs of the spontaneous abortion of a normal pregnancy following amniocentesis? The health service costs will include hospital staff, the use of a bed and operating theatre; the patient costs will include the avoided costs of a healthy child, plus the incurred costs of pain and suffering (for which the courts can provide some guidance on social judgements of financial value), as well as the time taken off work by the woman and the time spent by her family caring for her. Managers may well not feel equipped to judge the accuracy of costs presented in an evaluation; they should, however, demand a complete list of the assumptions which have been made, so that expert opinion can be sought as to whether or not the end result is likely to be acceptable.

Part of the argument will depend on what sort of costs have been used; the manager will have insight into the difference between fixed and variable costs. But costs also need to be comparable in other ways, particularly their interrelationships. Have the opportunity costs been similarly identified for everyone affected by an evaluative study? Is one cost marginal, another average total, another variable? Have all costs been discounted so that different expenditures at different points in time are expressed in a similar fashion?

Unless all costs are treated in the same fashion, they cannot be used to reach any conclusion in an evaluative study.

In economic terms, benefits imply the adding of value or the avoidance of payment. In assessing the benefits quantified in any evaluative study, the manager should check the following:

- exactly what is being quantified (effectiveness, utility or benefit);
- relevance;
- how values have been attached;
- clear differentiation from costs; and
- interrelationships (opportunity, marginal, time-scale).

Cost-effectiveness

Cost-effectiveness evaluations keep one side of the equation constant. Thus they can be used to compare the different costs incurred by using differing means to achieve the same end result. 'Effectiveness' is these studies is deliberately a limited concept, but still very useful. For example, there are different methods of attaining a given uptake of vaccination in young children: their parents can be sent appointments, health visitors could make home visits, or a van could visit given locations at set times. In each instance, the level of uptake may be similar. It is the costs which differ. An evaluation would not take into account other attributes of the end product, such as the opportunity to discuss child-rearing practice, or the attractiveness of attending for future vaccination; it would simply compare the different costs of the uptake of vaccination and immunization.

An alternative cost-effectiveness approach is to keep the cost constant and measure different outputs. A simple example would be cost and volume contracts – what variations in volume might a purchasing authority obtain for a given cost? Again this ignores other important dimensions, such as the quality of care which is purchased. Information from cost-effectiveness evaluations is very helpful, as long as their limitations are understood.

Cost-utility and cost–benefit

Cost-utility studies offer increased sophistication in the way the end result (the outcome or output) is measured; they acknowledge the complexity of any end result by, for example, quantifying how far a 'good' result in one dimension may compensate for a 'poor' result in another.

They still distance themselves from any judgement as to the 'worthwhileness' of an intervention; this is the arena for *cost–benefit analysis*. Measuring outcome and output is a difficult enough matter anyway; an awareness of the implied 'worth' of any activity, whether implicit or explicit, is an essential part of interpreting any of these studies. In addition, both sides of the equation – costs and benefits – may be different. The comparisons are more complex.

Assessing the relevance of an evaluation

The relevance of an evaluation can only be judged on an individual basis, but managers will need all their 'helicopter' talents to stand above a mass of detail and see what, if anything, contributes to local decisions.

The means by which values are attached to effectiveness, utility or benefit should be clear in any evaluation. What are the sources? How credible do you find them? What do you think they really mean? Does the process fit with your everyday understanding of the world? It is helpful to ask someone to say, out loud, in simple, monosyllabic English, what the implications are of each set of values used, not only on their own, but also in relation to each other. It is possible for some outcomes to have ten times the value of another, and not notice it in the calculations unless this deliberate 'walk me through it' approach is taken. For example, in the past, the average contribution of workers to the gross national product has been used as a benefit to justify the cost of treating renal failure; but what about high and low earners, women and children, the unemployed or retired? Another method, used in the calculation of QALYs assumes that someone confined to bed and suffering mild distress, is prepared to give up 44% of their life expectancy for a 'normal' life. Benefits, and their quantification, require imagination and intellectual rigour.

The effects of an intervention should be clearly differentiated from the costs. This may seem extremely obvious, but it is all too easy, for example, for savings in staff time to be hidden in the cost calculations, or for negative effects to be 'disappeared' because they are not to the liking of the evaluator. It should be possible to construct a clear table of costs and valued 'benefits', each of which may be positive or negative, from any evaluation with which you are faced.

The comment about interrelationships is the same as that for costs. Have opportunity costs been allowed for? Are these absolute or marginal benefits? Is everything in the calculation subject to the same time-scale?

QALYs: A brief outline

Another idea popularly associated with health economics is that of QALYs; they are a measure of cost-utility. The acronym stands for quality-adjusted life years. There are two main theses underlying the use of QALYs:

1. That for illustrative purposes, the quality of life can be represented in two dimensions (disability and distress).
2. That the treatment required to move from one level of distress/disability to another can be calculated.

The significant difference from other methods of 'valuing' health services is that this approach says 'yes, we can measure survival after an intervention, but the *quality* of that survival is also relevant'. So, if a person with a severe illness were only expected to live for 1 year without treatment but their survival were enhanced to five years, that would be one important part of the calculation; but we could also quantify what the quality of life in the single untreated year and the 5 years following treatment would be, and compare them. The calculation of QALY's includes:

- costs of treatment;
- changes in survival/life-expectancy;
- changes in quality of life (in two illustrative dimensions).

The summary figure (QALY) is the change in survival ('life year') reflecting the change in distress and disability ('quality adjusted'), i.e. the change in survival is weighted by a factor representing quality of life. Moreover, 1 year of full quality life is deemed equal to 5 years of one-fifth quality life.

Note that in the context of treatment of non-fatal diseases (e.g. artificial hip replacement for arthritis), it will be the duration of benefit from the procedure (e.g. average survival time of prosthetic hips) rather than that of the patient that figures in the QALY calculation.

Distress and disability

Research into possible methods of scaling levels of distress and disability was undertaken by researchers in the UK and the USA during the 1960s and 1970s, and an important publication in respect of QALYs was that by Kind *et al.* in 1982.[1] Seventy people were asked to score the levels of disability and distress in a complex sequence of questions. The median response was aggregated into a single matrix. The process is summarized in box 5.1 and the matrix portrayed in box 5.2.

The main features to be noted from the matrix, and which are crucial to an understanding of the QALYs are that:

1. The complete absence of any disability or distress is given a value of unity; anything less is a proportion of unity, and death is valued at zero.
2. It is possible to have a state worse than death – there are negative values.
3. The matrix can be utilized to calculate an 'exchange rate' between quantity and quality of life. For example, a person in disability category I, distress category C, would be prepared to trade-off [1 − 0.990 = 0.01 =] 1% of their life expectancy to achieve a state without disability or distress; and someone in disability category VII, distress category B, would trade-off [1 − 0.564 = 0.436 =] 43.6% of their remaining life expectancy in that state for 1 year with no disability or distress.

This foundation work has been severely criticized on three main grounds:

- the underlying philosophy;
- the methodology, because there was significant variation in the responses of these different groups comprising a small sample; and
- it is not clear that the sample is representative of the population at large.

Box 5.1   Assignment of scores to disability

The Scales

Disability
   I. No disability
   II. Slight social disability

   III. Severe social disability and/or slight impairment of performance at work. Able to do all housework except very heavy tasks
   IV. Choice of work or performance at work very severely limited. Housewives and old people able to do light housework only but able to go out shopping
   V. Unable to undertake any paid employment. Unable to continue any education. Old people confined to home except for escorted outings and short walks and unable to do shopping. Housewives able only to perform a few simple tasks
   VI. Confined to chair or to wheelchair or able to move around in the home only with support from an assistant
   VII. Confined to bed
   VIII. Unconscious

Distress
   A.   None
   B.   Mild
   C.   Moderate
   D.   Severe

The people asked

1. 20 healthy volunteers
2. 10 doctors sufficiently experienced to have gained a membership or fellowship of at least one college
3. 10 patients from medical wards
4. 10 psychiatric in-patients
5. 10 experienced SRNs (psychiatric)
6. 10 experienced SRNs (general)

What they were asked to do
1. Rank six 'marker states' in order of severity.
2. Place the six states on a scale, on the basis of 'how many more times more ill is a person described as being in state 2 than state 1' and so on. This was the most difficult aspect of the interview
3. Rank 23 further combinations of pain and disability
4. Express all 23 states in ratio terms including assigning 'one' to the state which it would be reasonable to restore all patients. The marker states could also be adjusted accordingly
5. The assumptions (as under 2) regarding prognosis were changed such that all states were permanent and hence not treated. Respondents were asked to adjust the scale accordingly
6. Place the state of death on the scale of permanent states, and assign a value to it

Box 5.2   The distress/disability matrix

Disability rating	Distress rating			
	A	*B*	*C*	*D*
I	1.000	0.995	0.990	0.967
II	0.990	0.986	0.973	0.932
III	0.980	0.972	0.956	0.912
IV	0.964	0.956	0.942	0.870
V	0.946	0.935	0.900	0.700
VI	0.875	0.845	0.680	0.000
VII	0.677	0.564	0.000	− 1.486
VIII	− 1.028	Not applicable		

Fixed points: healthy = 1; dead = 0.
Source: Kind *et al.* (1982).[1]

None the less, it has been the basis for considerably more work, and has stimulated some very important debate on the values which are used by decision makers about the use of health care resources. Fallowfield's[2] book contains discussion of the advantages and disadvantages of quality of life-scales.

Calculating QALYs

Conceptually, the costing part of calculating QALYs should be the easy bit. If someone is suffering a great deal of distress or disability, and a medical intervention claims to improve their quality of life, it should be feasible to cost that intervention and compare it with others. The calculations also take into account the life expectancy of the sufferer before and after the intervention; for example, renal transplantation can dramatically improve the quality of life of people with renal failure, but because the operation carries certain risks, particularly in respect of the drugs required to prevent rejection of the transplanted kidney, there are going to be differences in the pattern of survival for dialysed and transplanted patients.

Unfortunately, the calculation of QALYs founders upon major difficulties, including accurate assessment of the outcome data and of the costs.

There is a paucity of good, appropriate and usable health service evaluations. Relatively few health service interventions are thoroughly evaluated; even fewer have their evaluations expressed in terms of disability or distress. This is because the majority of clinical evaluations involve the simple survival/death dichotomy as an end point, or biological markers which imply but do not equate to the quality of life following an intervention.

This is a weakness of evaluation studies, not necessarily of QALYs, but it does imply that heroic assumptions sometimes have to be built into the calculations. Take the treatment of children with cancer as an example: biologically, the cancer may be eradicated, the proportion of children surviving 5 years with a treatment may be much higher than those without the treatment; but the impact of years of treatment on the quality of life will be significant, and there is an increased risk, it seems, of other cancers developing in some of these children as they reach adulthood, so that survival of the initial cancer by no means promises a normal life, nor a normal life expectancy. This does not mean that there have not been enormous advances in the treatment of children with cancer; but forcing the results into a two-dimensional matrix, no matter how sophisticated the trade-offs within that matrix, is a far from simple matter. All of the warnings raised in the previous section about understanding the measures of efficacy and benefit are pertinent here.

In addition, accurate and relevant costs of health service interventions are, or have been, extremely difficult to come by. This is largely because existing financial systems in the NHS have been designed to answer far more general issues (what does this hospital cost to run?) rather than specific queries (how much does the treatment of a heart attack cost?). One likely impact of the NHS and Community Care Act 1990 is that provider units will be required to develop increasingly sophisticated accounting systems to facilitate moves from block contracts to cost and volume contracts and, ultimately, individual billing arrangements. This detailed financial knowledge of case costs may, in turn, drive increasing demands for detailed evaluations of what the resources committed achieve in human terms.

Table 5.1   Comparison of costs per quality-adjusted life year (QALY) gained for various health care procedures, 1983–84 prices

Procedure	Value of the extra costs per QALY (£)
Pacemaker implantation for atrioventricular heart block	700
Hip replacement	750
Coronary artery bypass grafting (CABG) for main vessel disease	1,040
Kidney transplantation	3,000
Breast cancer screening estimated by working group to fall in this range	3,000–5,000
Heart transplantation	5,000
CABG for moderate angina with one vessel disease	12,000
Hospital haemodialysis	14,000

Source: Williams (1985).[3]

Despite these difficulties, some calculations have been made, and extensively used. They allow some sort of comparison of the relative expense and achievement of various health service activities (see Table 5.1). It can be seen that the calculation of QALYs, or any attempt to value the impact of health service interventions, brings together the skills of health economists and service effectiveness evaluators. The use of QALYs depends heavily on their skills, and also on the way in which resource allocation decisions are made (this aspect is discussed in more detail in Chapter 12).

Chapter 6

Descriptive, testimony, case studies and case-control studies

Introduction

In this chapter, we describe four of the most frequently encountered types of study. For each of them, the main advantages and disadvantages are listed, and these are then illustrated by drawing on published work. This is intended to be a very practical chapter – no single method is perfect, but we hope that the illustrations will provide a good feel for what it is like to undertake evaluative work of this nature, and that our readers will be encouraged to get involved themselves.

The appropriate selection of a type of study will also depend on the time-scale within which the evaluation is being carried out. This is illustrated in Fig. 6.1, which we feel is a useful summary to be borne in mind when reading the rest of this chapter.

Descriptive studies

Descriptive evaluations are very useful, especially for anyone who feels diffident about his or her skills as an evaluator. They can be done with relatively few resources, but at the same time require disciplined thinking and a clear structure, which is excellent experience for anyone wishing to develop their skills further. Their main features are some means of portraying a service, what it does and who does it. These studies also involve descriptions of why the service exists, i.e. what its main objectives are: this can be difficult to ascertain and set out clearly. Finally, they involve the evaluator's understanding of the context within which the service operates. No service is isolated from the rest of the world. The skill for an evaluator lies in understanding and focusing on significant relationships.

There are five main advantages of descriptive studies, and three main problems which need to be borne in mind. These are listed below. Three descriptive studies are then used to illustrate the points.

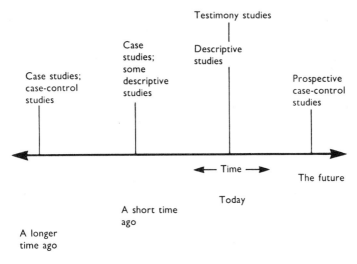

Fig. 6.1 Types of study and time-scale.

Advantages and disadvantages of descriptive studies

Advantages:

- They are possible with minimal resources.
- They involve service providers (thus 'ownership').
- The process of description can help clarify service objectives.
- They are repeatable, i.e. they can be used in times of continual change.
- The involvement of service providers enhances credibility, and thus facilitates management action.

Disadvantages:

- They require skills of observation and interpretation.
- They can appear 'soft' or 'unscientific' because they are not packed full of hard quantitative data.
- They may confront a manager with issues which he or she might prefer hidden, if he or she does not know how to deal with them.

Examples of descriptive studies

Illustrations are chosen from three studies: the first was published by the Social Services Inspectorate in 1986; the second and third were local evaluation studies undertaken in the North Western Region in 1989, one of which was to do with community-based health care provision and the other a hospital day unit.

The first was instigated in 1985 as a result of increasing public and professional concern about child abuse. In particular, it focuses on the supervision of social workers in the assessment and monitoring of child abuse when children subject to a court order have been returned home. The second describes the tentative development of a Chinese health information centre in Manchester city centre. The third is result of nursing staff in a surgical day unit documenting patients' satisfactions and dissatisfactions, and the actions which have been taken as a result. Their key features are summarized in boxes 6.1, 6.2 and 6.3.

In terms of resources used, none of these has made exceptional demands. No additional staff were employed. The first was undertaken as part of its general work by the Social Services Inspectorate. The second was largely the result of work done by a trainee in public health medicine, very committed to the concept of the Chinese Health Information Centre (CHIC), who worked with her colleagues at the centre in putting together the evaluation. The third, initiated because of the concerns of nursing staff, was carried out by those nurses and was acted upon by their managers.

This last also emphasizes how descriptive studies can involve local service providers, who thus contribute considerably to their commitment to improving and developing the services where they work. The evaluation report of the CHIC was checked and rechecked with the staff working there, so that it was perceived as both 'fair' and accurate, and as a result the recommendations were also acceptable and eminently feasible.

The Social Services Inspectorate met initially with the senior staff in each social services department, and then with middle managers, and practitioners,

---

Box 6.1   An assessment of monitoring procedures for child abuse

Inspection of the supervision of social workers in the assessment and monitoring of cases of child abuse when children, subject to a court order, have been returned home.

Objectives :
1. To investigate current social work practice and to identify methods of good practice which can be disseminated by the Department
2. To produce a report which could be the basis for a self-inspection format
3. To identify any implications for the training of social workers and their supervisors

Undertaken by:
Social Services Inspectorate

Method:
Comparison of observations against standards of good child care practice encapsulated in *aides-mémoire* specifically prepared for the study

Outcome:
A Guide for Social Workers undertaking a comprehensive assessment,[2] published 2 years later

---

Source: Social Services Inspectorate (1986).[1]

Box 6.2   Chinese Health Information Centre (CHIC) Evaluation 1987–89

Purpose of the evaluation:
1. To assist in planning
2. To provide information for funders
3. To stimulate interest in the work of the CHIC
4. To provide feedback to staff

Undertaken by:
Senior registrar in community medicine (public health medicine), a research nurse, a nurse co-ordinator and a general practitioner

Method:
Combination of financial and activity data, group discussions with staff (agreeing the centre's aims and objectives), discussions with users, and consumer questionnaires and checklists

Outcome:
Widespread demand for report; invitations to address seminars in the North West and elsewhere; used by Regional Group for Black and Minority Ethnic Groups

---

Source: Chinese Health Information Centre (1989).[3]

Box 6.3   Day surgery service effectiveness study: Preston Health Authority

Objectives (implied):
1. To encourage health service staff to evaluate their service
2. To measure aspects of the service thought to be inadequate
3. To provide pointers for action to improve the service

Undertaken by:
Nursing staff in day surgery unit

Methods:
Questionnaire developed and analysed

Outcome:
Improvements to the service: environment (ward temperature); discharge policy; staff rotation to keep knowledge up to date; further work on the areas of patient care

---

Source: Welton and Barker (1989).[4]

individual supervisors and social workers. The result is a detailed and prescriptive guide for social workers undertaking a comprehensive assessment. It is unlikely that any guide could have been published, certainly not in so much detail, had it not had its origins in the day-to-day details of social work.

The pragmatic nature of the report was also due to its clarifying the service objectives. The inspectors made their evaluation against a standard of good child care practices using *aides-mémoire* compiled as a result of consultation with experts in practice, supervision and management, including representatives from the voluntary sector and social work education. Clear aims and objectives were perceived as particularly important by the CHIC, since they not only provided a background against which evaluation could take place, but also provided a clear explanation and purpose for essential supporters and funders. The general concerns of the day unit nursing staff were expressed very clearly in the forms of questions they identified for patients using their unit.

Repeatability only seems relevant for our two local examples. The CHIC certainly perceived evaluation and objectives as integral and evolving, rather than rigid and unreactive. Similarly, the questions developed in the day unit are being used repeatedly to assess whether or not the desired changes have been successfully implemented and are also being enhanced to address other issues which are being raised.

We have already commented on the importance of the involvement of service providers and how this has enabled management action. This is, perhaps, particularly striking in the case of the day unit, where it is quite obvious from reading the reports that not only did the nursing staff feel an obligation to assess what their patients thought of the unit, but the managers also felt an obligation to take action on what their nurses discovered. This action has included clarifying and implementing a discharge policy; converting changing rooms to more private facilities for examination and history taking; and effective means of monitoring environmental temperatures.

It is, as one would expect, less easy to detect some of the difficulties involved in descriptive evaluations from published reports. Generally, only those evaluations which have managed to overcome the difficulties will reach the public domain. However, it is worth noting the skills which must have been needed in the Social Services Inspectorate report, where it is apparent that, at times, extensive efforts had to be made to understand exactly what had happened, particularly in respect of the 'gloomy' state of much information recorded on children's files. The inspectors point out how social workers often attached considerable significance to the change in an isolated factor relating to a child, and as a result accorded less significance to continued factors that still remained a significant part of that child's environment. Skills, experience and understanding are essential in a report of this kind, enabling the investigators to point to the significance of the lack of information regarding male figures in the home, the absence of details regarding the criminal activities of family members, and the lack of recognition by some practitioners of the importance of evaluating the relationship between the child and his or her parents.

Considerable skill was also needed in the evaluation of the CHIC, because this document not only identifies key objectives for the centre, but also represents the broad agreement of at least a dozen or more staff about the key topics to be addressed in such a report, and how they should be looked at. Perhaps less skill was needed in asking the right questions in the day unit evaluation, although the very positive use of that evaluation and of the issues it raised, in itself requires managerial skill.

It was also possible for the two local studies to quantify a considerable amount of their evaluation, whether it was the number of patients who raised a particular issue, or the proportion of individuals attending the CHIC who came from different parts of Manchester. The Social Services Inspectorate deals far more in generalities. For example, there are unquantifiable statements: 'a lack of clarity was surrounding the position of level 3 social workers ... there was confusion about ... supervision or consultation ... managerial or professional'. There is, however, no doubt at all about the practical significance of the problem identified and this sense of reality must be worth a great deal whenever any sort of behavioural change is envisaged.

Finally, none of the reports identifies issues which managers cannot cope with. They are all very positive and foward looking. However, one of the issues identified by the Social Services Inspectorate was the inability of social work managers to make productive use of a review system which they should already have been undertaking. The detailed nature of the guidance published subsequent to this research could only be of help to those managers.

Doing descriptive studies yourself: Some hints

Bear the following points in mind when embarking on descriptive studies.

1. Do talk to a number of people involved in the service before you start (it is often helpful to list the key players, and add to the list as your contacts increase).
2. Do write down on paper your ideas of the main aims and objectives of the service and discuss these with the people you meet.
3. Do find out what data are routinely collected by and concerning the service.
4. Do look up relevant literature and published guidance.
5. Do decide from whose perspective you particularly wish to describe the service.
6. Descriptive studies can be an exciting way of integrating evaluation with the provision of a service. They do not need to be written in purple prose, but the ability to communicate clearly is essential for their success. So, finally, do set out enough time to sort your thoughts out and decide what you want to say, to whom you are saying it, and the best way to make sure you get the message across.

Testimony studies

Testimony studies may be used to describe a service, but they are also an evaluative methodology in their own right. They involve the deliberate selection of people from whom testimony will be sought, the decision about whether to seek this testimony from individuals or groups, and a means of recording all that is said and making some sense of it afterwards. Perhaps more than any other type of evaluation, they require the researcher to be very clear at the outset about the likely biases which may come up as a result of using this method – considerable preparatory work is needed. But more than that, they also need the evaluator to be able to hold the fine balance between preventing his or her own prejudices from blocking off what the witnesses are saying at the same time as exercising sufficient discipline to keep the collection of information structured, relevant and focused on the issues in question. This can be a dangerous tight-rope. It is possible to identify six key advantages to this evaluative process, but also six problems of which the practitioner should be aware.

Advantages and disadvantages of testimony studies

Advantages:

- They can be very rich in ideas and ways of dealing with a situation.
- They provide a valuable basis for detailed work.
- They can provide very rapid information (no need to await complex data analysis).
- They make it possible to probe immediately for detailed and underlying understanding.
- They can be particularly relevant where behaviours are being evaluated.
- They encourage participation in evaluation by individuals who may not be particularly literate.

Disadvantages:

- Skills are required to encourage testimony.
- They may be best when performed in groups, and these may be difficult to organize and manage.
- Recording all that this said and the way it is said (verbal and body language) is difficult.
- There may be difficulties in interpreting and understanding what is said.
- No statistical quantification is necessary, and therefore they may appear 'soft'.
- They may be very difficult to repeat.

Examples of testimony studies

Two examples have been chosen to illustrate the power and pitfalls of testimony evaluations. The first documented the use of focused group discussions to evaluate health promotion campaigns related to AIDS, as a result of the perceived inadequacy of conventional quantitative methods. The second was undertaken for the NHS training authority and is one of a series of management studies, where testimony has been collected from NHS managers, a 'new breed' with the introduction of general management into the NHS. There was a general need for this relatively new concept to be studied in sufficient detail for its practitioners to learn from their peers' pitfalls, techniques, anxieties and

---

Box 6.4 Exploring young people's attitudes to and knowledge of AIDS: The value of focused group discussions

Objectives:
1. To assess awareness of AIDS and HIV-related disorders and concern about them in relation to other health issues
2. To assess reactions to media campaigns
3. To elicit participants' predictions about their sexual behaviour in the future
4. To assess the use of discussion as a means of exchanging information between peers and as a forum for promoting changes in attitude

Method:
Focused group discussions

Outcome:
Part of accumulating evidence, that many recipients of the AIDS campaign did not identify with it, leading to suggestions for more specific and targeted approaches.

Source: Boyle *et al* (1989).[5]

Box 6.5 Templeton series on district general managers

Objectives:
1. To understand the DGM's job and identify the strengths and weaknesses of different approaches
2. To shed light on the key issues for effective management in the NHS
3. To draw lessons which will help in the selection, development, evaluation and performance of general managers

Methods:
Tracer study over 2 years of 20 DGMs involving quarterly interviews supplemented by frequent discussions in between

Outcome:
Study folders published by NHS Training Authority; recommendations acted upon by NHS Training Authority

---

Source: NHS Training Authority (1987).[6]

progress. The details are given in boxes 6.4 and 6.5.

Both studies are rich in ideas, e.g. the moral stance displayed by some members of the AIDS Group: 'AIDS is killing off the weak ones.' The Templeton study was able to document the ideas which district general managers had for involving doctors in management (building up close relationships with key consultants; developing networks which link them into the power groups; furthering individual doctor's special contributions; and demonstrating the usefulness of general management).

Although neither claims to have been the basis of further detailed work, it takes little imagination to see how the AIDS study could be used to structure a closed questionnaire regarding attitudes to AIDS advertising, and one of the authors of this book is using the Templeton study as one source from which to develop further research of doctors in management.

Both papers are excellent examples of the rapid production of information. The AIDS study was published within a year of its commencement. The Templeton study lasted 2½ years, and published issue papers throughout that time.

The opportunity to probe was actually part of the group behaviour recorded in the AIDS study, where participants corrected each other's misapprehensions about AIDS and about 'safer sex'. The Templeton study is an excellent example of how testimony can expand on the sort of general statement which is quoted in its introduction:

> ... unless managers get the doctors with them, everything else is just window dressing. That's where you have got to get to change ... there will never be a better time.

Both papers relate to behaviours – the first to sexual behaviour in the light of an intense health promotion campaign, and the second to behaviours in the light of intense management pressure.

However, neither of these two papers required the involvement of non-literate individuals. This does not mean it is not still a valuable advantage of the approach. For example, the Health Education Authority, in developing a new campaign aimed at improving vaccination and immunization uptake, specifically involved people from lower socio-economic groups, where uptake is known to be much lower. The focused group is a traditional evaluation technique for marketing.

As regards the disadvantages of testimony studies, it is not evident from the papers that there were problems to get the participants to talk. This is hardly surprising, given that the group in the AIDS study were undergraduates starting a degree in psychology, and in the Templeton study they were senior health service managers. However, in the latter, the research process involved lengthy quarterly interviews, with frequent telephone conversations in between, and sustaining sufficiently good relationships with busy and stressed individuals over 2½ years sufficient to be able to continue collecting data requires particular skill.

It would certainly be interesting to know how much more the Templeton study might have achieved had it been able to bring together some of the managers in groups, so that they could bring out ideas in one another. The AIDS study had little difficulty with this, because it was undertaken using local students. However, the selection of individuals to join a group, the size of the group, the environment, and upon completion of the group work to leaving all participants with the feeling of having made a positive contribution, has to be managed as professionally as any other research approach.

As regards recording the testimony, neither study identified difficulties, but it takes little imagination to think through situations where it might prove virtually impossible to document all that is going on. The same applies to interpreting and understanding what was said, and for the AIDS study it would also have been necessary for the researchers to have a detailed knowledge of AIDS. And the statement by one consultant involved in the Templeton study ('Thank God we didn't get someone from Sainsbury's) was perceived as part of a common assertion by many working in the health service that it is something special, and not susceptible to a managerial or commercial approach. Thus, skills are needed, not only to record what is said but its underlying meaning too.

Neither study had any statistical quantification and both studies were particularly relevant to the time when they were done, and thus extremely difficult to repeat.

As the health service becomes more managed and more 'consumer aware', the use of testimony studies may become increasingly relevant. As already mentioned, this is a time-honoured marketing approach. There is little doubt that in the future we are going to have to develop a deeper understanding of what our 'customers' think of our marketing attempts in respect of, for example, cervical screening and family practitioner brochures.

Doing testimony studies yourself: Some hints

Bear the following points in mind when embarking on a testimony study.

1. Do be particularly clear about your aims and objectives – once you start collecting testimony, it may be difficult to change.
2. Do consider carefully how the testimony will be recorded; it may be helpful to work with a colleague.
3. Do pilot the study. Piloting is always important, but especially so if the researcher's personal listening and probing skills are at risk of being exposed. If you are having the testimony collected by someone else, be very clear about what you hope to glean.
4. Do grasp opportunities to probe what the witnesses are saying – there is an immense wealth of information to be collected this way.
5. Generally, this technique is stimulating and can be exciting; it can also be exhausting. Do ensure that your witnesses feel that you are all ears *for them*.

Case studies

Testimony studies tend to be dynamic 'action research', and their reports are very much the result of an interaction between the researcher and the researched. There are times when it is necessary for someone trying to evaluate service effectiveness to stand back, to take the broader view, and too see if it is possible to put some boundaries around and some shape into a particular issue.

Case studies have always formed part of the traditional medical approach to understanding disease. For example, reports of individual cases with unusual presentations are making us aware of the very wide ramifications of child abuse[7] where, in clinical terms, an individual case is assumed to have an important contribution to make to our understanding of the wider issue of child abuse. In the same way, the case study which is to be used as an illustration of evaluating service effectiveness attempts to throw light on a broader issue by looking in detail at one case. In this instance, we have drawn on a US study, where the authors examined the effect of the Medicare prospective payment system on the adoption of new technology by studying the case of cochlear implants (see box 6.6).

Box 6.6   The effect of the Medicare payment system on the adoption of new technology, in this instance cochlear implants

Objectives (implied) :
1. To describe an underfunded but effective technology
2. To compare payment with cost
3. To describe the history of use of cochlear implantation
4. To ascertain rationing of the availability of the advice

Methods:
Determination of costs and payments for the service

Outcome:
The case study concluded failure of widespread adoption (and subsequent consortium of manufacture) due to financial disincentives

---

Source: Kane and Manoukian (1989).[8]

Above all else, a case study involves a clear working hypothesis, a belief that a set of circumstances (or symptoms, or physical characteristics) can be explained as an example, a 'case', of a more general phenomenon. The evaluator thus needs to have some familiarity with the general phenomenon, be it a particular disease or a management process. It is also necessary to have enough specific facts so that the example (i.e. the case) is clearly defined and understood, and can be related to the general phenomenon. Because doing this is such a useful and educational discipline in itself, case studies are frequently used to help students understand a general lesson they have been taught. In the same way, a case study can provide salutary information for service evaluation.

The advantages and disadvantages of case studies

Advantages:

● They require little in the way of resources.
● They can provide a good way of building a body of knowledge.

- As a means of understanding situations, they fit comfortably in a tradition of medical and social sciences.

Disadvantages:

- They are generally only applicable to individual patients, organizations or situations.
- The definition of what comprises a suitable case may vary, thus making comparisons over time virtually impossible.
- By relying on the skills of the observer, interpretation may be heavily biased.
- They generally do not allow a statistical analysis.

Case studies need not involve much in the way of resources if one thinks in terms of personnel alone. For example, in the same issue of the *New England Journal of Medicine* that published Kane and Manoukian's article, the average number of authors per article was 6.6; Kane and Manoukian make only two.

By focusing on one particular technology, they have expanded our knowledge about the impact of a restricted prospective payment scheme so that we are forced to recognize that financial considerations may far outweigh clinical desires, and that if there is no demand in a market economy, manufacturers go out of business. The approach is one which can be understood by both managers and clinicians. It is also one of the measures which may be used in clinical audit, an educational tool of increasing importance.

Although in this example the resources used in terms of personnel were few, a great difficulty with case studies is the ability of the student to project the lessons from the specific case onto the broader canvas. And, as Barbara Stocking[9] describes in her study of innovation in the NHS (*Inertia or Innovation*), it can be very difficult to have a clear definition of what comprises a suitable case. More than ever, the value of this particular technique depends very much on the skills of the researcher to see beyond the immediate example and identify implications for health services as a whole. There is no doubt that their interpretation can be biased by, for example, political or clinical interest.

Statistical calculations may not always be possible, although in the case study used as an example, the authors were well able to quantify 'underpaying DRGs' and the differential in cost and reimbursement for cochlear implants.

Doing case studies yourself: Some hints

When embarking on case studies consider the following points:

1. Do clarify your hypothesis before you start – what is it the case study shows?
2. Do check your interpretation of events – you may have missed something or misjudged something seriously.
3. Do make sure you have documented all the salient facts – make a very long checklist and keep updating it.
4. Do keep asking yourself 'so what' as you write – a case study can be thought of as a piece of a jigsaw, so help it fit the awkward space.

Case-control studies

One of the problems of case studies, useful as they are, is the discipline required for structured thinking about an issue. For the readers of such studies, it can be difficult to prove or disprove the assertions and interpretations which are made. Unless there is some means of comparing cases which share all but a few key characteristics, it is impossible to judge, in any quantified manner, the real impact of those key qualities. Case-control studies provide a means of getting round these difficulties. They have an honourable history in epidemiology as a means of testing hypotheses about the cause of disease (e.g. smoking and lung cancer; exercise and mortality from heart disease). They are also an excellent means of quantifying the impact of an intervention.

As the name implies, this sort of study involves groups (sometimes matched pairs) of subjects: 'cases' and 'controls'. The study design is based on the common notion of *cause and effect*. It is assumed that the presence of a specific characteristic is likely to lead to a particular outcome (and hence to a *case*) and that absence of the characteristic, in subjects similar to cases in other respects, is less likely to lead to the outcome. In contra-distinction to the intervention approaches outlined in Chapter 7, case-control studies start with subjects to whom the outcome *has occurred*, i.e. cases, and look into their histories to find the prevalence of characteristics which it is thought may have caused that outcome; for comparison, a control group to whom the outcome has *not occurred* is examined in the same way; if the prevalence of the putative causative characteristic (or documented event) is *greater* in the case group than in the control group this supports (but does not prove) the notion that a cause and effect relationship existed. Subjects may be persons, services, institutions etc. Figure 6.2 portrays the essential difference between case-control studies and intervention studies.

The main skills required for doing a case-control study are (1) the skill of defining precisely what the specific characteristic is and (2) the skill of matching cases and controls as perfectly as possible in every other important respect. Considerable knowledge of the topic being evaluated is required. Moreover, it is advisable to seek statistical advice when designing and analysing case-control studies.

The advantages and disadvantages of case-control studies

Advantages:

- They should minimize bias.
- They should thus maximize learning.
- They should be statistically robust.
- They should be repeatable.
- Of all the techniques mentioned so far, the case-control study is the only technique by which any sort of causal relationship can be imputed.

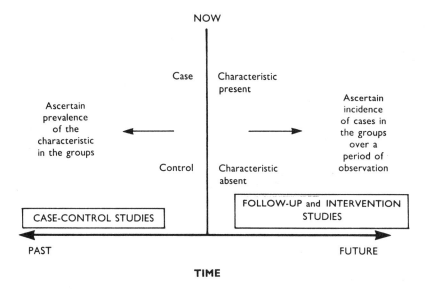

Fig. 6.2 Case-control and follow-up studies.

However, see the discussions in Chapters 7 and 11 on the imputation of cause.
- They are not as costly as intervention studies.
- An answer is usually obtained sooner than from an intervention study.

Disadvantages:

- It can be extremely difficult to avoid bias.
- It can be difficult to achieve sufficient numbers.
- It can be expensive compared to the other approaches discussed in this chapter.
- They require meticulously detailed documentation and analysis.
- They cannot give as strong an imputation of cause as intervention studies.

Examples of case-control studies

Three papers have been selected to illustrate case-control studies. The first is the more traditional 'causal' approach, but particularly interesting for managers, since it relates to the reasons why patients are not admitted to hospital. The second was stimulated as a result of awareness that the residents of a large mental handicap institution seemed to be suffering from hypernatraemic dehydration (a potentially lethal condition) and studies its prevalence, and then monitors a change in prevalence following intervention, using the case-control technique. The final example also relates to evaluating the effectiveness of a preventive strategy: bicycle safety helmets and the severity of head injuries suffered by cyclists. Boxes 6.7, 6.8 and 6.9 illustrate their key features.

Box 6.7   Non-admission or non-invitation? A case-control study of failed admissions

Objective:
To examine the causes of non-admission to hospital

Methods:
1. Examination of medical records
2. A questionnaire given to non-attenders (cases) and attenders (controls)

Outcome:
Despite a common tendency to blame patients for non-admission, factors due to patients are fairly unimportant

---

Source: Frankel *et al.* (1989).[10]

Box 6.8   Hypernatraemic dehydration in patients in a large hospital for the mentally handicapped

Objectives:
1. To determine the prevalence of hypernatraemic dehydration
2. To assess the hydration and nutritional state of patients in a large hospital for the mentally handicapped
3. To assess the efficiency of an intervention programme

Methods:
The blood sample and body mass index of patients in a large hospital (cases) were compared with those in a small hospital for the mentally handicapped (controls)

Outcome:
New nursing procedures were introduced into the large hospitals, thereby preventing the hypernatraemic dehydration that was associated with previous nursing practice

---

Source: MacDonald *et al.* (1989).[11]

Minimizing bias is an extremely important part of a case-control study. By prejudicing the inclusion or exclusion of certain groups for an evaluative study, for example, may prejudge the issue so much that the evaluation is, in effect, worthless. For example, in the case of non-admission to hospital, a testimony study might simply have revealed the prejudices of those interviewed, that problems were largely due to patients simply not turning up. By looking in detail at the records for admitted and non-admitted patients, and by sending a questionnaire to a sample of each, the first study was able to show quite clearly that in only a tiny proportion of cases (1–3% of all booked admissions) did

---

Box 6.9   A case-control study of the effectiveness of bicycle safety helmets

Objective:
To quantify the effectiveness of bicycle safety helmets in preventing head injury

Methods:
The clinical details of cyclists attending emergency departments with head injury (cases) were compared with cyclists attending the same departments with other injuries (controls) and cyclists reporting any accidents (additional controls)

Outcome:
Bicycle safety helmets are highly effective in preventing head injury, particularly for children

---

Source: Thompson *et al.* (1989).[12]

non-admission occur without prior notification (by the patient) to the hospital. In addition, because admitted and non-admitted patients were similar in many respects, they were able to emphasize the importance of the procedure (varicose veins were associated more with non-admission and hip replacement with admission) which, of course, may be due either to medical or patient factors.

This means there is a very clear lesson to be learnt from this paper, as was also the case in the study of hypernatraemic dehydration. By comparing the residents of one institution with those of another, and the residents of the community, the authors were able to show quite clearly that the residents of one institution were at far greater risk than those elsewhere.

The statistical robustness is particularly important where any intervention is recommended. The purchasing and wearing of a bicycle safety helmet may appear to be a relatively trivial intervention, but it is one of a number of medical pronouncements on life-style and, as such, justifies serious evaluation before it is widely broadcast. In addition, because this was a large study, the authors were able to explore and control for other salient factors, such as age, sex, income, education, cycling experience and the severity of the accident. They found riders with helmets had an impressive 85% reduction in their risk of head injury and an 88% reduction in their risk of brain injury.

It would be possible to repeat all three studies and, in fact, the study of hypernatraemic dehydration reports case-control studies repeated after an intervention.

The major strength of case-control studies is that it is possible to impute a causal relationship: that hospital organization factors contribute significantly to the non-admission of booked patients to hospital; that mentally handicapped residents of a large institution need not be at high risk of hypernatraemic dehydration if the staff ensure that all residents consume adequate quantities of fluid and do not use hypertonic enemas; and that bicycle safety helmets are highly effective in preventing head injury. It is of interest to note that in certain states in Australia, it is now a legal requirement for cyclists to wear a helmet.

However, the power of this evaluation is bought at a price. Controls and cases have to be carefully selected to avoid bias. As an illustration, it would not have been as helpful if the study of hospital admissions had explored non-admission in patients attending one speciality and admission in patients attending another, since this would obviously make considerable difference to their age, sex and social circumstances.

Larger numbers also make statistical analysis easier, but it may not be possible to recruit them. In the study of hypernatraemic dehydration, there were less than 100 residents as cases and only 50 controls from another institution. Considerable statistical expertise is needed to aid the interpretation of any changes in the context of relatively small numbers.

Obtaining the numbers, and the statistical expertise, can be expensive. The study of the effectiveness of bicycle safety helmets was based on five major hospitals over a 12-month period, and involved collecting data on over 1200 patients altogether.

The data on all these patients will have had to be meticulously detailed, standardized and documented to allow, for example, regression analysis to control for age, sex and other factors. The discipline which is needed to achieve this is extremely important. It is all too easy to assume that all participants in a study understand what is meant by commonly used words like, for example, 'high blood pressure'. A properly conducted case-control study would ensure that there is a clear definition of all terms used.

Case-control studies can be held up to be an excellent means of demonstrating health service effectiveness in any evaluative study. However, they are only one of a number of approaches, all of which contribute to both managerial and clinical understanding.

Doing case-control studies yourself: Some hints

Consider the following points before embarking on case-control studies:

1. Do assemble a good team to help you before you start. As a minimum, you are likely to need expert help with knowledge of the topic under investigation, with statistics and with computing.
2. Do be very clear about the source of any information you intend using to describe the cases or controls, let alone any intervention or outcome. How good are the data? Is the quality of data likely to prejudice or impair your study?
3. Do set aside enough time and enough resources; case-control studies are very rewarding but very demanding. The rigour of this study design has to be paid for.
4. Do check again and again that the cases and controls are well matched. Suspect bias in everything. Otherwise your painfully achieved results may be ridiculed because someone else spots something you had not considered.

Chapter 7

Intervention studies

Introduction

Intervention studies are the most powerful means of evaluation. They entail making deliberate changes to procedures or services and studying the consequences. Thus, the possibility of an intervention study arises when someone suggests that a change to the structure, organization or content of a service will confer benefit.

Before an intervention becomes plausible, there has to be a theoretical understanding or hypothesis about the relationships between the entities under study and of what the nature of the outcome of the intervention might be. Therefore, intervention studies should be well-designed experiments to refute or confirm benefits which have been supposed before the study is undertaken. The importance of clearly articulating the theoretical context within which *any* study takes place has been mentioned in Chapter 2 and will be discussed further in Chapter 11.

The power of intervention studies flows from the attempt to alter (or intervene in) chains of cause and effect. Showing that altering an assumed cause brings about a change in its putative effect (e.g. clinical outcome) is *direct* evidence that the cause and effect relationship exists. Knowledge of particular cause and effect relationships confers power to manipulate the world around us, e.g. to effect successful treatment of some diseases.

Intervention studies do not differ in intent from the techniques discussed in Chapter 6. Indeed, all the methods discussed in this book are elaborations upon the definition of evaluation in Chapter 1. However, whereas the methods of Chapter 6 (e.g. case-control studies) are often capable of giving strong evidence that a treatment or service does or does not meet its aims, such evidence is nevertheless indirect or circumstantial. It is only the intervention study that is capable of providing direct evidence. Even so, it is very difficult to construct intervention studies on human populations or institutions that have the potential rigour of laboratory experiments and in which factors extraneous to those under study are wholly controlled. Also, intervention studies are expensive, difficult to conduct and usually require a fairly long time-scale. Thus intervention studies are best reserved for circumstances where alternative approaches are *a priori* inadequate or, having been tried, are inconclusive and the consequences of a wrong decision would be costly.

Sadly, it is not difficult to find examples of medical practice being uncertain through a lack of suitable intervention studies or the picture being confused through inappropriately designed ones. An instance of each will suffice to make the point.

The treatment of chronic ear infection in very young children is a contentious area of practice. It is claimed that children who develop glue ear may suffer retardation of language development and, in addition, some fairly uncommon long-term physical sequelae have been documented. The insertion of grommets (tubes) to provide drainage from the aural cavity via the ear drum is a plausible procedure which is in wide use.

The grommets remain in place for a few weeks or months before dropping out. Alternative treatments using antibiotics and/or steroid drugs have been suggested, as has the combination of surgery and drug therapy. While there has been a number of clinical trials – some being of elegant design – the issue of treatment has not been resolved because the trials do not address themselves to the long-term outcome for the child. Little is known about the natural history of chronic ear infections in children and neither has this been related to long-term language development or the effect of any of the possible therapeutic interventions. In the meantime, while knowledge remains uncertain, medical practitioners can justify, on largely anecdotal evidence, whichever treatment regimen they wish. The insertion of grommets takes up much of the time of ear nose and throat surgeons in the NHS and in private practice. It has been suggested[1, 2] that the preoccupation with grommets is a means of filling the gap left after childhood tonsillectomy and adenoidectomy operations became unfashionable.

The cause of neural tube defects, such as spina bifida, is a mystery. In the 1970s, there was considerable effort to seek environmental and dietary agents which might explain variations in the occurrence of these congenital anomalies. Epidemiological evidence[3] pointed to vitamin deficiencies in mothers during the early stages of pregnancy as a possible cause. In consequence, Smithells and colleagues[4] undertook a trial of periconceptual vitamin supplementation in women known by virtue of previous neural tube defect births to be at high risk.

The findings from the study, if taken at face value, indicated that vitamin supplementation was beneficial. The study aroused great public interest. Unfortunately, the subjects in the trial had not been randomly allocated to treatments (see next section) and the authors had overlooked a number of very serious sources of possible bias to their findings; these were rapidly pointed out in the medical press. However, this study, which can be described as inconclusive, has made it difficult to settle the issue by a randomized controlled trial. Some doctors began prescribing vitamin supplementation and also women could buy vitamins freely from chemist shops. Indeed, some people, who clearly cannot have understood the nature of the evidence, argued that a further trial would be unethical as this would entail withholding possible benefit from some women. These matters greatly hampered the Medical Research Council in its attempts to sponsor a conclusive clinical trial.

The notion of levels of evaluation introduced in Chapter 2 is applicable to intervention studies. They may be applied to individual treatments (e.g. one technique *vs* another) or to services (e.g. breast screening). They may be applied to procedures targeted at individuals or those targeted at defined populations (e.g. health promotion campaigns). In general, the further one moves from the individual procedure applied to the individual person, the more difficult it becomes to design and execute an intervention study. Moreover, the further one moves from individuals, the more likely that serious methodological compromises (e.g. definition of comparison groups) will have to be made, and in consequence the intervention study may give rise to evidence as circumstantial in nature as that from the methods discussed in Chapter 6. Even so, at this level it is often feasible to design worthwhile intervention studies. A clear understanding of the methods involved and of the biases to be controlled aids the decision as to the best way to proceed.

Randomized controlled trials

In introducing intervention studies, we begin with the potentially most rigorous approach – the randomized controlled trial (RCT). The first proper RCT is credited to a study of streptomycin in the treatment of pulmonary tuberculosis conducted by the Medical Research Council in 1948. Sir Austin Bradford Hill was a leading promoter of the early trials and contributed much to the subsequent development of the technique. A brief history of the RCT may be found in Pocock.[5] Latterly, Professor Archie Cochrane[6] was a major exponent of the RCT and he aroused much ire within the medical profession when he rightly pointed out that most of the then, and now, current clinical procedures had never been properly evaluated and were of unproven worth.

The use of RCTs has become increasingly common in the evaluation of clinical procedures aimed at individuals and it can, in principle, also be applied to services as a whole and mass health promotion activities. With respect to clinical procedures, use of the RCT is not restricted to complicated or expensive treatments; it is being applied to the evaluation of nursing practice and diverse examples[7-11] of this use may be found from any scan of the recent literature. Many other examples of RCTs are cited in Pocock's book.[5]

An understanding of the principles of the RCT is essential not only to those planning to undertake one, but also to those having to make service planning judgements on the basis of clinical trials. Clinical procedures of proven efficacy should be the bedrock upon which services are built. Moreover, the evaluation of the effectiveness of overall services (e.g. breast screening), rather than individual procedures, must take place on the assumption that the procedures (e.g. radiographic technique and treatments for early breast cancers) which contribute to the service are of known efficacy; in these instances, the would-be investigator should first have looked critically at the evidence supporting this assumption. Moreover, an understanding of the counsel of perfection (the RCT) assists investigators to assess the impact of biases consequent upon being forced to depart from perfection.

The following discussion of the RCT is an introduction to concepts. There are many technical ramifications upon which we will not dwell. Some material is recommended in the Further reading list. However, anyone embarking on a RCT should also consult a medical statistician.

Randomized controlled trials: The basics

A simple instance of a RCT would be as follows. A team of investigators wish to compare the efficacy of two drugs denoted as treatments A and B. These drugs will be used in the treatment of a common cancer (e.g. lung cancer) and the measure of outcome will be how long patients survive after being recruited into the trial.

Upon diagnosis, the eligible patients will be informed of the purpose of the trial and asked to consent to take part. Those consenting will then be *randomly* allocated to either treatment A (the current best drug) or treatment B (a new drug). They will receive their treatments (which in all probability will be a lengthy course) and the investigating team will keep track of each individual's survival. After, say, 3 years, the investigators will calculate the proportions of patients surviving each course of treatment and compare the results. On the basis of this comparison, they will conclude which, if either, was the most effective treatment. If one treatment was demonstrably the better, the investigators will quantify the degree of benefit. The key features of this *grossly* simplified account are:

1. A comparison is made, in this case between two groups. This is a feature of all evaluative work, and is stressed throughout this book.
2. Random allocation to the treatment groups.

In the absence of a comparison group of patients, there would have been no standard against which to judge the efficacy of the new drug; the nomenclature of RCTs uses the word 'control' to denote a baseline comparison group.

But why randomly allocate; wouldn't 'picking' two similar groups of patients do, or could one allocate patients alternately to treatments? First, let us be clear what random allocation means. In this instance, a random allocation entails each patient having a one in two (or 'fifty-fifty') chance of being allocated to either treatment and that chance being in no manner altered consciously or unconsciously by the preferences of doctor or patient or by any other extraneous circumstance. Thus the random allocation is *as if* for each patient a fair coin had been tossed and heads means treatment A and tails treatment B. Under this regimen, patients with various characteristics that might alter their response to treatment are distributed evenly between the treatment groups. It is assumed that these are underlying biological or social characteristics which are not yet known to medical science as prognostic factors or which, if known, the investigators do not feel the need to take formal account of in the design of their study.

Any method of allocation which is not strictly random is always open to the suspicion that some factor, known or unknown, may have led to one group of patients differing in important characteristics from the other and that this may have influenced the observed effect of the treatment. To take an extreme case, if the investigators attempted to allocate patients haphazardly, but not strictly randomly, their decision might unconsciously have been influenced by their judgements of the severity of disease; the more severe might, say, have ended up on the new treatment, which naturally the investigators believe to be a 'wonder drug'.

It is more difficult to pin down what is wrong with allocating patients alternately to treatments. But there is always the suspicion that a systematic method of allocation might somehow end up synchronized with some biasing factor that determines the order in which patients reach the investigators' consulting room door. For example, an out-patient sister may, without being conscious of it, alternate severely ill and not so severely ill patients when organizing the order in which they see the doctor; her motive is humane and understandable – she wishes to spare the doctor from seeing *all* the most severely ill patients one after another. But if the doctor were innocent of what she was doing to relieve his stress, he might unwittingly ensure that only less ill patients were selected for the new drug – and of course they would seem to do much better than the others. Proper random allocation is straightforward and is discussed on pp. 162–4.

It should be noted that randomization only takes place *after* the patients have consented to participate. Those patients who are prepared to be involved in research may differ in a number of relevant aspects (e.g. psychological, social and physical) from those who do not give consent. Explaining the process of randomization or the 'fifty-fifty' chance can be difficult, particularly if the investigator is prejudiced in favour of one treatment or another. However, the concept can be grasped, and must be discussed with the patients before randomization takes place, or there is a very serious risk of the results being biased.

Biases and other problems

The findings of a RCT such as that portrayed above should not be taken at face value. The investigators and those subsequently acting on the findings of the study must satisfy themselves that bias was eliminated and that the study was inherently capable of providing the answers sought. The issues to consider include:

1. Whether the diagnostic criteria for patients entered to the trial are clearly stipulated and could be replicated by others.

2. Whether the treatment regimens are clearly stipulated.

3. The degree to which it is possible to extrapolate from the findings on the particular patients entered into the trial to ordinary medical practice in those specialities which might be applying the results. This is an important point, because patients entered into clinical trials tend to be a highly selected subset of all patients with the same disease. The selection factors include:

- patients in trials often attend specialist centres to which referral sometimes depends upon the severity of disease;
- the entry criteria to trials are often, and quite reasonably, tightly drawn so that the patients being studied are a homogeneous group;
- there are often strict exclusion criteria, i.e. patients with particular complications or other current disease will be excluded because these factors might make interpretation of the findings of the trial more difficult; and
- patients who consent to take part in trials do not necessarily respond in the same way as those who withhold consent.

Thus, it is sometimes found that applying the findings of promising trials to the generality of patients encountered in ordinary medical practice proves less beneficial than was anticipated.

4. Although the random allocation of patients to treatment groups offers the prospect of distributing patients with hidden prognostic factors equally among the groups, it gives no guarantees. It is in the nature of chance events that unbalanced patterns will occur by chance alone. However, the larger the numbers of patients in the treatment groups, the less likely that gross imbalances will occur. Furthermore, the larger the number, the more likely it is that the patients will represent the range of hidden prognostic factors to be found in the generality of patients to whom the trial's findings might one day be applied.

The problems considered here can be handled in two ways. First, if there are known prognostic factors (e.g. age, gender or ethnicity), the trial might be designed as a series of sub-trials. That is, patients may be randomly allocated to treatment groups *within* their prognostic categories (e.g. allocate males and females separately). This is known as pre-stratification.

The second approach, which may be used in conjunction with pre-stratification, is to look at the distributions of measurable characteristics among the patients within the treatment groups when the trial concludes. If these are found to be grossly unbalanced (e.g. more smokers in one group than the other), then during the analysis the patients can be subdivided within the treatment groups by the characteristic of interest and the analysis conducted as a comparison between the treatments *within* characteristic groups. This is known as post-stratification. Obviously, nothing can be done in the case of characteristics which have not been measured or in the case of unknown prognostic factors.

5. A trial which is too small is incapable of giving a definitive finding. This

is an issue separate to that mentioned in 3 above. It is common to all studies, not just RCTs, and will be discussed on p. 169.

6. Biases can arise through the expectations of doctors, nurses and patients if they know which treatment a patient is receiving. This can work in subtle ways that are not well understood. However, it is widely accepted that a patient's psychological state influences physical response to treatment. Thus if patients believe they are receiving a 'wonder drug' or are expected to do well they may – for reasons unconnected with the efficacy of the drug – fulfil the prophecy.

These biases may be eliminated through making people 'blind' to what is going on. Thus, in a *single-blind* trial, the patients are not aware of which particular treatment is being administered. In a *double-blind* trial, neither the patients nor their daily carers are aware of which particular treatment each patient is receiving. Obviously, this is only feasible when the treatments are administered in the same manner (e.g. tablets) and can be disguised (e.g. by the pharmacy) to look alike.

A third refinement is the *triple-blind* trial, wherein the investigator doing the statistical analysis of the trial is unaware of which treatment was which, i.e. he or she has access only to codes. This eliminates any possibility of an investigator's expectations unconsciously influencing the way the data are handled, and leads to less temptation to make special pleading for inconclusive patterns in the data which appear to bear out the investigator's expectations.

7. In a trial of long duration, bias can arise through incomplete follow-up of patients. Patients may move away and perhaps become untraceable. If, for instance, the end-point measure of the trial is life or death, then it is possible that some of the terminally ill may cease to attend follow-up clinics or indeed move away to die in peace. The problem is what assumptions to make about missing patients (i.e. those whose fate is unknown). There may be equal numbers of missing patients for the two treatment groups, but one treatment may have been so poor that all the missing people are dead, whereas the other was so good that all the missing people have joyously gone off to lead a new life. The only solution to this problem is to maintain rigorous follow-up, which might also entail keeping track of death certifications through national agencies (e.g OPCS in the UK).

Related to this is the adequacy of duration of follow-up. The duration must be long enough to give good prospects of encountering the expected benefits and any major hazards. If remission of disease is a major end-point measurement of the study, then the follow-up period may have to be many years.

8. Some therapies give rise to adverse reactions or other sequelae which mean that the therapy has to be stopped and another substituted. In the context of a clinical trial, this means that the patient will cease to be receiving the treatment originally allocated. If in any of the study groups withdrawals from treatment are frequent, this poses difficulties for those interpreting the trial. It

is widely accepted that to analyse a trial *as if* withdrawn patients had never been included in the first place, is totally unjustifiable and may give rise to serious bias. The best practice is to include all patients entered in the trial and follow all up until the end of the trial. During analysis, all of the patients – regardless of how their treatments may later have altered – are considered to belong to the treatment groups to which they were originally allocated. This is known as *analysis by intention to treat*. All the main conclusions of the trial should be based on this analysis. However there is nothing to stop investigators looking at their data in other ways, but these further analyses should be regarded as informal and the findings as suggestive rather than definitive.

9. Whether the end-point (outcome) measures of the trial were appropriate to the kind of use to which one would wish to put the findings of the trial. This will be discussed in greater detail below.

Further elaborations of the RCT

The trial discussed above was very simple but it did encapsulate the main features of a RCT. However, clinical trial technology has advanced tremendously and there is a variety of variations on the basic theme. Some of these relate to the design and others to statistical analysis. We shall touch on a few of these. RCTs are able to compare more than two groups, but unless a factorial design is used (see below) it may be difficult to recruit sufficient patients.

It is unnecessary for all of the treatment groups to be involved in active treatment. Sometimes there is no current best treatment with which to compare the new treatment or we may suspect that current treatments are useless and wish to confirm this. In these cases, it is prudent, if practicable, to give the 'no treatment' group a dummy treatment (e.g. an inert drug). This dummy, known as a *placebo*, ensures that any difference found between the 'no treatment' and 'active treatment' groups is not attributable merely to the psychological *placebo effect* of the active treatment but represents a genuine effect. The placebo effect should not be underrated: it underpins (at great cost for useless treatments) much of modern medicine.[12]

The numbers of patients in the different treatment groups (*arms*) of a trial need not be equal. Indeed, if there has been true unrestricted random allocation they are unlikely to be. However, the point being made is that sometimes issues of statistical precision may lead investigators randomly to allocate, say, twice as many patients to one treatment arm than to another.

Many diseases are too uncommon for it to be practicable to recruit an adequate number of patients for a study of reasonable duration at one centre; hence the multi-centre trial. These may involve collaboration between many centres in several countries. Single-centre trials can be costly and difficult to organize and these problems compound in multi-centre trials. A multi-centre trial requires a detailed protocol to which all participants agree to adhere. It is particularly important that all centres follow the same diagnostic criteria, recruitment criteria, treatment regimens, procedures for measuring end-points and follow-up practices. To keep such an enterprise on track and to ensure that the findings are recorded and collated, a trial co-ordinating office with experienced staff is required. An excellent example of a multi-centre study which the reader might care to examine is the Medical Research Council trial on the treatment of mild hypertension.[13,14] A particular problem those investigators had to face was standardizing the manner in which the collaborators measured blood pressure. It should never be assumed that because a technique is in common use, people do it in a way which meets the rigorous requirements for consistency demanded by a study.

Sometimes it is possible to increase the statistical precision of a trial without having to increase the number of patients. For instance, in certain skin conditions or illnesses which effect both of a pair of organs (e.g. ears), it may be feasible to treat differently different parts of one patient's body. Thus each patient is entered into both treatment groups of the study simultaneously. In essence, each patient is their own control and the study consists of many replicates of simple experiments on separate people. An illustration of this approach may be found in a report from the Diabetic Retinopathy Study Research Group[15] of a trial in which photocoagulation treatment and non-treatment were randomly assigned to the eyes of individual patients. The reason why this procedure increases precision is explained in Chapter 11.

A variant of the foregoing is the cross-over design. This is applicable when the subject's response is being studied over a fairly short period of time. It may be possible to give each subject two different treatments one after the other and compare the responses to each. Subjects would randomly be allocated as to which of the treatments they receive first. An amusing example is the study by James *et al.*[16] on the effect of oxprenolol on stage fright in musicians.

Another elaboration involves what are known in statistical parlance as factorial designs. These involve subjects receiving various combinations of different treatments which could in some instances be combinations of surgery and drug therapy. A particular feature of these designs is that they enable investigators to examine the effects of treatments separately and in combination; the combined effect may be more (or less) than the sum of the individual effects – a phenomenon known as synergy to pharmacologists and interaction to statisticians. These designs can also increase precision. A detailed account of factorial designs is given by Cochran and Cox[17] and for an illustration of their use in a clinical trial see the study by the Canadian Cooperative Study Group[18] on the effects of aspirin and sulphinpyrazone in threatened stroke.

The analysis of the end-point measures in our simple example (treatments A *vs* B) above was naïve. We assumed that the investigators would merely compare the proportions alive and dead in the two groups after 3 years. In real life, it is to be hoped (sometimes vainly) that the investigators would avail themselves of statistical techniques of survival analysis which look at the patterns of survival throughout the course of the study and not just at one point. Extensive information on this and other matters pertaining to lengthy trials is to be found in two excellent articles by Peto and colleagues.[19, 20]

In our simple example we assumed that the investigators would run their trial for a fixed time and then analyse the results. When it can be expected that the response to treatment will occur shortly after the treatment (days rather than months), is is feasible to collect the outcomes as the trial proceeds. Successes and failures can be observed to accumulate for each treatment. There may come a point at which so many successes accumulate for one treatment that it is felt that these are sufficient evidence that the treatment is the better and that the trial should stop. Indeed this has two advantages: a trial can cease engendering unnecessary further cost; it is ethically desirable as soon as possible to cease subjecting patients to treatments proven ineffective. This approach has been formalized and made statistically respectable and such trials are known as *sequential clinical trials*. However, in practice, there are fewer opportunities for applying this technique than might be hoped. For further information on this approach, the reader is referred to Pocock.[5]

Many trials have multiple-outcome measures, not all of which need be clinical. Indeed, as shall be mentioned later, this is highly desirable. Nevertheless, multiple measures can be difficult to interpret and put towards an overall view about the efficacy and desirability of a treatment. These are issues to which thought is best given at the design stage of a trial rather than having to make sense of a morass of data at the end.

Our discussion, being primarily concerned with the science and technology of RCTs, has avoided ethical issues. These are important and, in particular, the question of what constitutes informed consent to enter a trial is not resolved and practice differs between countries. An introduction to these considerations and a portal to the wider literature is provided by Pocock.[5]

The remainder of the discussion of clinical trials will concentrate on general rather than technical matters. And, finally, other ways of using the RCT will be examined.

What should RCTs of clinical efficacy accomplish?

Drug drials are often classified into the following four categories, which correspond to stages of experimentation:

1. *Phase I trials*. These are concerned with drug safety, pharmacological action and optimum dose levels. They are small-scale in nature and usually involve healthy human volunteers. Efficacy is not at issue at this stage. These trials are usually the responsibility of the manufacturer. They are not RCTs.

2. *Phase II trials*. These are small-scale trials on carefully selected patients who are monitored in detail. The aim is to establish the plausibility of efficacy and detect drugs whose side-effects outweigh their possible benefits. Ideally, these should be RCTs but phase II trials are not always this rigorous. These trials usually require close collaboration between the manufacturer and a clinical team.

3. *Phase III trials*. These are large-scale comparisons of new drugs with existing treatments. They are the only source of convincing evidence that a new

treatment confers benefit to the generality of patients for whom it is intended. In our opinion, phase III drug trials should *always be RCTs*. Furthermore, although it is desirable that manufacturers should fund phase III trials it is, in our opinion, essential that the trials be supervised, analysed and written up by independent investigators.

4. *Phase IV trials*. These are concerned with the surveillance of morbidity (e.g. side-effects) and mortality once a drug has been licensed for general clinical use. They are necessary because although a well-designed phase III trial will be capable of establishing whether or not a treatment has efficacy and whether there are any gross side-effects, it is unlikely that the numbers in the study will be large enough for the detection of rare side-effects; moreover, many phase III trials are of too short duration to detect side-effects consequent upon prolonged use of a drug. These observational studies are sometimes organized by the manufacturer. However, in the UK, there is a Department of Health sponsored 'yellow card' scheme whereby practitioners report to a central monitoring unit any suspected adverse reactions.

The schema outlined above can be carried over to any clinical research on efficacy, e.g. to studies on surgical treatment, screening modalities and diagnostic procedures. Phases I and II correspond to initial small-scale studies which in many instances may be fairly informal. On the basis of these, investigators may be able to formulate a convincing argument that the circumstantial evidence of benefit justifies the costs and risks of an extensive RCT (phase III). Phase IV then corresponds to the monitoring that should be applied to any procedure in routine use.

Within this context, the purposes of RCTs become clear. They can be any of the following:

1. *To question the assumption that an unevaluated treatment, which is in routine use, confers benefit.* Many trials have been undertaken with this intent and often surprises have ensued. A notable example was the Northwick Park electroconvulsive therapy trial[21] which greatly clarified the clinical indications for this kind of therapy and knowledge about the duration of benefit. In most instances, the results of such trials show either that efficacy has been grossly overstated and/or result in more precise indications for when treatment is likely to confer benefit.

2. *To evaluate a new treatment which theoretically offers tremendous benefit.* When coronary bypass surgery was first introduced, the potential 'market' of eligible patients was believed to be so large that health planners in the UK were concerned that demand for treatment would outweigh any affordable hope of meeting it. A series of clinical trials[22, 23] clarified the picture greatly: it was shown that those most likely to benefit were people with intractable angina or three-vessel disease. Moreover, the benefit in terms of improved life-expectation was quantified.

3. *To evaluate a new treatment which promises to be less costly or less hazardous but not necessarily more clinically effective than an existing*

treatment. In this instance, an RCT would be designed to demonstrate that the new treatment has not unacceptably less efficacy than existing ones.

Outcome measures in RCTs

RCT technology was developed to help clinicians ask critical questions about their clinical procedures. Naturally, the questions asked have tended to be clinical in nature, e.g. how long does remission last, what is the length of survival, what degree of pain relief is attained? All of these can be quantified and all fall within the domain of the clinician's experience. However, there are two reasons why this simple clinical approach is inadequate to present needs.

1. It is becoming increasingly recognized that what the clinician deems as success or failure does not necessarily correspond with the perceptions of the patient and the patient's family. Particularly in chronic disease, which forms the major burden of illness in the community, questions of quality or life loom larger than merely biological indices. Of course pain relief, for example, is an aspect of quality. But quality of life has many other facets connected with independence, freedom from the burden of long-term drug intake with invariable side-effects (why else do so many hypertensives fail to 'comply' with treatment?), and the patient's own perception of the relative benefits of short-term life-quality compared to long-term gains.

Consider the treatment of small cell lung cancer. This disease is almost invariably fatal within 5 years and the vast majority of patients are dead within 2 years. Clinical trials abound and their end-point measures are primarily tumour regression (strictly an end-point for phase II trials) and survival. The treatments, standard and new, are always unpleasant and offer little benefit to the patient. Almost invariably these trials make no attempt to measure the patient's perception of quality of life. Ten years ago, this criticism might have been unfair because quality of life is extremely difficult to measure convincingly. However, there has been a great deal of work by psychologists and sociologists and credible measuring instruments have emerged.[24]

2. Because health care resources will always be finite, there is an implied rivalry among patient care groups and among the care options within these groups. Thus, if those who are to make choices on behalf of the community are to do so rationally, they must have information about the cost, cost-effectiveness and cost–benefit of treatment options (see pp. 68–75). This information is difficult to obtain merely through observing current practice or through studying the reports of traditional clinical trials. However, it is relatively straightforward to build in an economic component when designing a phase III trial.

The upshot of the foregoing remarks is that clinical trials should not be seen as the exclusive domain of clinicians and statisticians. They require collaboration with medical scientists, psychologists, sociologists and health economists. Furthermore, the content of proposed clinical trials is a legitimate concern of health care planners and managers. These are matters that funding bodies, ethical committees and the higher reaches of health management should pursue.

A broader use of RCTs

The discussion of RCTs has concentrated on instances when the object of study has been the responses by patients to treatment. In statistical parlance, the *study units* were individual people. Also, the example of an RCT (see pp. 95–7) can loosely be thought of as the many-fold *replication* of a simple trial involving one case and one comparison. The concepts of study unit and replication apply to most evaluative techniques and they will be further discussed in Chapter 11. Here, however, the notion that a study unit is an individual will be relaxed.

The study units in a RCT can be groups of individuals or institutions. For instance, two health promotion techniques applicable to workplaces may be compared. The study units will be workplaces and the outcome of the trial some measures of the impact of health promotion on *groups* of people, e.g. proportion ceased smoking for a year. In designing this trial, one would seek to select a 'population' of workplaces which was fairly homogeneous with respect to size and nature of industry. The workplaces would randomly be allocated to the alternative health promotion campaigns.

The principal determinant of the power of this study to discriminate between the hypotheses under test (e.g. which technique best reduces cigarette smoking) is the number of workplaces, i.e. 300 workplaces of 50 employees each gives a much more useful study than 50 workplaces of 300 employees each. This is because the outcomes are being measured on workplace response rather than individual response.

The bare bones of this design could be elaborated upon to include a number of sub-studies which look also at smaller groups of people within workplaces and perhaps at individual responses to some interventions. However, if it is necessary to look at individual responses it should be remembered that the responses within a particular workplace are likely to be correlated; this is a consequence of the workforce having something in common. Thus, all analyses of this trial which seek to make comparisons between subgroups of people should make those comparisons *within* the workplaces. It would not be acceptable to pool people between the workplaces as that would entail combining like and unlike.

Sometimes – as for example in the evaluation of a screening service – it would be desirable to allocate individuals on a random basis to receive and not receive the service, but it may prove unacceptable to design a study on this basis. An alternative is to provide the service on an all-or-none basis in different geographical areas and then on a random basis to allocate the service among the areas. The study units are now geographically defined populations and the outcome measures might be the incidence of disease or mortality statistics for those areas.

Spurious alternatives to the RCT

RCTs are difficult, time-consuming and expensive to conduct. Furthermore, some moral philosophers have gone so far as to suggest that the random allocation of patients to treatments is unethical; we regard such arguments as mischievous. Nevertheless, there are grounds for seeking simpler alternatives. It is probably not practicable to subject all unproven procedures in current use to RCTs, although we believe that all new procedures, particularly those with large costs (financial to the NHS; pain, inconvenience or life-style disruption to patients), should be so subjected. We shall outline some alternatives and see how they measure up to the 'gold standard' of the RCT.

Historical controls

It is sometimes argued[25, 26] that instead of using a comparison group of randomly allocated current patients it will suffice, if due care and attention is taken, to use the records of patients who have previously been treated with the comparison therapy; these patients are known as *historical controls*. The mainstream of opinion is *firmly against* the use of historical controls: there is no way of being sure that like is ever being compared with like. Indeed, the literature contains interesting examples[27, 28] of the wrong inferences which can arise from the use of historical controls; the evidence points to the biases in patient selection leading to conclusions more strongly in favour of new treatments than would be the case from comparable RCTs.

Incidentally, it should be clear from the discussion on pp. 97–100 that the preceding point is (if the word 'ever' is omitted) also strictly true of RCTs. However, any particular RCT is more likely to be unbiased if the treatment groups are large and, moreover, RCTs *on average* are unbiased as a consequence of the statistical properties of random allocation. An interesting discussion of historical controls may be found in Pocock.[5] As he says, on occasion historical controls may give an unbiased result but there is no way of knowing which occasions those are.

Clinical audit

Clinical audit was introduced in Chapter 4. It is a technique used by medical and paramedical professionals to subject their practices and those of their immediate colleagues to constructive criticism. Audit is an evaluative tool and undoubtedly will have an impact on quality of care. Although we cannot advocate it as a substitute for RCTs when new procedures are introduced, it nevertheless will be helpful in weeding out some current practices of doubtful validity. Also, issues explored during audit may sometimes be found to justify more rigorous examination by RCT. At least audit and the clinical databases, mentioned below, do not lull investigators into believing – as is the case for advocates of historical controls – that their studies have the power and precision of RCTs.

Clinical databases

Some centres routinely maintain *detailed* and *systematically* gathered records of the diagnoses, treatment and outcome of patients under their care; over the years, the number of records for a particular disease may become huge. These records, particularly if stored on a computer, are amenable to many interesting analyses. It is possible to *explore* how outcome alters according to differences in patient characteristics and clinical management. These insights may sometimes be sufficient to justify small changes to practice without recourse to formal trials. Jennet,[29] a leading advocate of the use of clinical databases, suggests that they may pose a challenge to RCTs; we remain sceptical. We follow Temple[30] in asserting that database analyses must be followed by trials.

Mathematical models

Jackson[31] describes mathematical modelling thus:

> The modelling approach to evaluation consists of considering an environment as it is found; of establishing its important features; of producing an idealization of the relationships between them, and then constructing mathematical equations to describe them. The mathematical equations when calibrated on a given set of data, form the basis for predictions of the future, or evaluations of the past or present.

Through examples, Jackson demonstrates the power of this technique. He contends that mathematical modelling is a substitute for RCTs even in circumstances when an RCT would be practicable.

Modelling is useful not least because it forces assumptions about and understanding of the system under review to be made explicit. Also, it is consistent with our predilection (see pp. 145-6) for developing theoretical frameworks as the context within which research takes place. Undoubtedly, well-formulated and robust models allow the exploration of issues difficult for RCTs to tackle. Nevertheless, as is accepted within the mainstream philosophies of science, theory and models have to be juxtaposed with reality through *experimental* test of their predictions. That is, a scientific theory, as distinct from a myth, has not only to explain some aspect of how the world of our experience works but also to enable us to predict the consequence of certain actions (or interventions); if those predictions are found to be untrue, then doubt is cast upon the theory. Experiment entails deliberately setting up the starting conditions (i.e. interventions), from which particular predicted events should follow, and observing the consequences.

Modelling, analysis of clinical databases and audit techniques are inherently non-experimental because they involve no planned and controlled intervention in presumed chains of cause and effect *which have not yet happened*. That is, the starting conditions from which the observed events flowed were not the consequence of a deliberate intervention by an experimenter.

Nevertheless, while denying that the supposed alternatives can ever have the power of the RCT, we do accept that they are useful for *fine-tuning* clinical knowledge and that they can explore some issues to which the RCT is unsuited.

Other intervention studies

A problem encountered when evaluating the effect of changes to entire services, e.g. the organization of a hospital's surgical unit, is that it may be difficult to identify one comparison service let alone to replicate the comparison. Furthermore, at the level of entire services, as distinct from their component procedures, random allocation often becomes unwieldy.

Thus there is sometimes a choice between doing no formal randomized experiment or of relaxing some of the standards of perfection. Pragmatically, it is usually better to do the latter but with full awareness of biases that could lead the findings astray.

Natural experiments

Natural (or opportunistic) experiments arise when some change to a service will take place anyway and investigators latch onto this in an attempt to answer questions on their own agenda. The example below is from epidemiology rather than health service research, and is based on work published by Thomas and colleagues.[32]

During the 1970s, there was controversy about the effects of lead on the development of children. Lead is not a natural part of the human diet and its main sources of entry to children is through the inhalation of car exhaust, ingestion of old-fashioned lead-based paints, certain cosmetics used by Asians, and drinking water. Lead is never present in water in the public distribution system but, particularly in soft water areas, it leaches out of the lead water piping found in some older houses. The question at the time was the relative contributions of the various sources of lead to the lead content of children.

Thomas *et al.* were interested in the importance of water-borne lead. Clearly, it would have been expensive, impracticable and unethical to set up a true experiment in which households were randomly allocated lead and copper piping. Fortunately, there were two council-owned housing estates of similar character, and close together in North Wales, one of which had copper household water piping and the other lead. The town council planned to replace all the lead piping with copper.

The 'experiment' consisted of taking regular tap water samples from the households on both estates. Blood samples were taken from mothers and children on the estates before and after the lead piping was removed. It was found that the tap water lead content was zero on the copper estate and moderately high on the lead estate. Moreover, the average blood lead levels were appreciably higher on the lead estate. After the lead piping was replaced with copper, the blood lead levels on the lead estate rapidly declined until they did not differ from that on the copper estate. The investigators were able to conclude, among other things, that ingestion of water by households with lead piping does contribute measurably to the body burden of lead.

This example illustrates two features which can make the findings of a natural experiment convincing. First, on the lead estate there was a *before and after* comparison; a change in blood (and water) lead was demonstrated to follow the intervention. Secondly, there was an external comparison – the copper estate in which nothing changed and in which the outcome measures did not alter. The lack of change in outcome in the comparison estate makes it more plausible that the changes in the lead estate truly resulted from the intervention and were not some mere correlate with a coincidental temporal effect.

Non-randomized controlled studies

If the random allocation of study units (e.g. people, hospitals, areas) to intervention and comparison groups is impracticable, then the best that can be achieved is to try to make the study units in the groups being compared as alike as possible with regard to important characteristics. This general approach is known as *matching*.

Matching may be done either between individual study units or, less rigorously, so that the overall distributions of characteristics in the groups being compared are similar. To make it more specific, consider a study in which there are two groups to be compared and in which the study units are individual people. Also, bearing in mind our strictures against non-randomization in studies on individuals given in the previous section, let it be assumed that to randomize is genuinely impracticable. The potential candidates for each group are assumed known.

Paired matching would entail selecting someone to join the intervention group and then seeking from the list of potential candidates for the comparison group someone who was, say, of the same gender, age, occupation, ethnic group, etc. The matching characteristics are chosen on the likelihood of them influencing the outcome. Obviously, the more factors there are to match, the harder it becomes to find suitable pairs. If the study units were institutions, the matching criteria might include size, location, nature of population served, organizational features, etc.

Group matching entails trying to ensure that overall there are similar proportions of people in various age bands, similar proportions of different occupational groups, etc., for each comparison group. There need be no particular similarity of characteristics of pairs of individuals chosen haphazardly from the intervention and comparison groups.

If paired matching has taken place or if the design of the study has involved any other kind of pre-stratification (cf. pp. 97–100), it will be necessary to take this into account during the analysis of the data. Such matters are beyond the scope of this book.

Strategies for service interventions

This section concentrates on studies in which there is a change to the organization or balance of a service and when an RCT is either not feasible or the nature of the answers being sought do not justify the time and expense. Such might be the case when the managers of a health district wish to evaluate a local change but are not seeking 'hard scientific' evidence of success with which to impress the rest of the world.

Three approaches are possible:

1. Compare the changed service with an unaltered one elsewhere. Better still, look for several comparisons matched to the service to be altered. This lessens the chance of the findings being grossly biased by an inappropriate comparison.
2. Compare the changed part of the service with another part of the same service which remains unaltered. This is feasible when the service is spread geographically over an area controlled by one health authority. For example, in an attempt to improve immunization uptake, a new method of follow-up of non-attenders may be introduced in some clinics and not in others. As always, try to compare like with like.
3. Do a *before and after* comparison. This entails taking the current outcomes as the standard for comparison with the changed outcomes after the intervention has had time to work. Clearly, this is even better if combined with method 1 above (cf. pp. 108–9).

The following issues should be taken into account:

1. The end-point (outcome) measures have to be carefully chosen. They have to be recorded in a standard manner and it is particularly important to check whether relevant information will be available if the comparison is with a service elsewhere. Sometimes, routinely available information may suffice.
2. The evaluation should be planned before the change is made. Only then will it be possible to ensure that relevant information is available for collection.
3. As far as possible, extraneous factors that might influence the outcome should be kept constant. This is a fundamental principle of all experimentation. Even when these factors cannot be controlled, they should be recorded. During interpretation of the results, some judgement will be required as to how far, and in what direction, extraneous factors have had an influence.
4. When changes have been extensive it may not be possible to unravel which elements of change had the main impact. This may not matter too much if the result is an improved service, but if there has been no impact on outcome it should not be inferred that each of the individual changes was ineffective: deleterious effects may have balanced improvements.
5. Lack of replication poses problems (see Chapter 11).

Chapter 8

Assessing patient satisfaction

Introduction

The 1983 Griffith Report[1] charged the then management board of the NHS with the following task:

> To ascertain how well the service is being delivered at local level by obtaining the experience and perceptions of patients and the community: these can be derived from CHCs [community health councils] and by other methods, including market research and from the experience of general practice and the community health service.

As is clear from this statement, it was envisaged that this task might be tackled in a variety of ways and through various agencies. In part, it can be approached as a general quality of care issue through the setting and monitoring of standards for hotel services, reception procedures, waiting times, front-line staff behaviour, complaints procedures, etc. Up to a point, routine monitoring can take place without the direct cooperation of patients and clients (consumers). However, the choice of standards should take account of the expectations and requirements of consumers, and not merely reflect professional views. Moreover, it is prudent periodically to ascertain that the findings of routine monitoring procedures are in accord with the actual perceptions of consumers. In general, the ways of accomplishing this are as follows:

- being receptive to anecdotal evidence;
- frequency and substance of complaints;
- frequency and substance of compliments;
- case studies;
- commissioned market research; and
- in-house surveys.

These will be discussed in the following sections; the greatest attention will be paid to in-house surveys.

Before proceeding, it is useful to remind ourselves of some of the factors which might influence people's feelings of satisfaction:

- staff approach and attitudes, e.g. the feeling that the consumer comes first;
- quality of information received on what to do and what to expect;
- appointments procedures;
- waiting times;
- general facilities on-site;
- hotel facilities for in-patients, e.g. quality of food, privacy and visiting arrangements; and
- outcome of treatment/care received.

It should be borne in mind that the aspect of quality which is uppermost in the professional's perception, namely quality of outcome, may not be the factor which most influences the consumer's feeling of satisfaction. Usually, the consumer, through lack of the necessary technical knowledge, is not in a strong position to judge the quality of the outcome; it is taken on trust. Also, any attempt to assess patient satisfaction and evaluate efforts at improving quality of care must be preceded by an analysis of which aspects of quality are being judged.

Finally, bear in mind that patient satisfaction is a true outcome measure of health services. It complements technical outcomes such as would be measured by efficacy or effectiveness. It is influenced by service *process* (cf. Chapter 1).

Anecdotal evidence

Anecdotal evidence is based on what people say during their ordinary social contacts with others about a hospital, a service, etc. Those expressing the view may or may not have actually experienced the service in question. Such evidence represents the casual, but sometimes heart-felt, view of the 'punter' in the street. It can be a true or false impression of the service; however, even in the latter case, it is important because it reflects feelings and attitudes in the community. For instance, of a major hospital in Wales the following has been heard to be said by an elderly woman with a condition requiring minor surgery: 'I wouldn't go into the XYZ because most people who enter there leave in a box.' This individual's perception of the hospital was partly true, but she had drawn a false conclusion with respect to her own risk of dying: the hospital receives a large number of acutely ill elderly patients of whom a substantial proportion die; given the case-mix the mortality is no more than to be expected.

Anecdotal evidence is sought by keeping one's ears open; it can be refined by the more formal techniques to be discussed below. It can be the starting point for informative detailed enquiry.

Complaints and compliments

Complaints and compliments can be informative. They both represent the tips of icebergs; i.e. they are brought about by people strongly moved to raise a voice. If the findings of complaints procedures are collated, it may be possible to discern patterns and trends. This information can be used as an outcome measure for an evaluation of a change in the way services are delivered. However, the fact that complaints appear to diminish in number or magnitude does not prove that a service has improved; people may no longer bother to complain because it appears to be of no use; the mass of little niggles which do not cross the threshold for formal complaints may in fact have increased.

Compliments are hard to assess formally. However, they should be fed back to the appropriate staff. Everyone appreciates encouragement.

Case studies

The contribution of case studies to evaluation is discussed on pp. 85–7. In the context of assessing patient satisfaction, the case study approach is useful because it allows an in-depth exploration of matters of quality of service which large surveys cannot accomplish. The findings of case studies should not be extrapolated in a quantitative manner to populations of consumers. Nevertheless, they do identify issues worthy of investigation by other means.

Market research

Market research has been used in commerce for decades. It is only recently that it has been applied to the NHS. In commerce, many large organizations have their own market research departments and their own fieldworkers; others use professional agencies. Manufacturers often wish to know who is buying their products, and what they think of their quality, their presentation and their price. Such information is used in their forward planning.

A good example of market research relating to a public organization is BBC audience research. In 1936, the BBC set up a listener research department now called, since the advent of TV, the audience research department. Each day a national quota sample of 2250 men and women are asked what programmes they viewed or listened to on the previous day. From these data, audience listening figures and viewing figures can be computed and producers use this information to plan times for future programmes. This market survey is complemented by getting the opinions of volunteer panels of some 6000 viewers and listeners. Volunteers are a self-selecting group and to get public opinion some form of survey or poll has to be undertaken. There are ways of sampling a population (see pp. 164–9) and certain organizations are skilled in their use. For instance, the Gallup organization often conduct pre-election polls and *Gallup poll* has passed into the English language. Other organizations well known in this area are Marplan Harris International Opinion Polls Ltd and Opinion Research Centre. Their methodology could be applied to obtaining and assessing patient opinion about the health service. Obtaining opinions may on first sight appear deceptively easy, but in fact there are many traps for the unwary which must be avoided if high-quality data applicable to the population as a whole are to result.

Conducting a patient satisfaction survey

Patient satisfaction with a service is one measure of outcome. An improvement in patient satisfaction over time could indicate improvement in the service. Intra-district comparison could be used as a performance indicator, a low ranking suggesting that there is further room for improvement and that such improvement is possible. Data on patient satisfaction can be obtained by postal questionnaires or by interview. The following issues must be considered.

1. *Planning a survey.* The first step is to state clearly the objectives of the study; the mere act of doing this will help to clarify the purpose of the survey in the surveyor's mind (see Chapters 2 and 3). Having set the objectives, the plan is then directed to achieving them with the required accuracy and within a given level of resource and a given time-span. It is then necessary to consider coverage. For instance, how is the population to be studied delineated? Is it by geographical, demographic or other boundaries (e.g. attenders of a particular clinic)? Arising from this are a number of subsidiary questions such as how the sampling should be done and what size of sample should be used. At this stage, it is important to consider the question of non-respondents and what action should be taken in dealing with them. Unless one is a competent statistician, it is important to consult a statistician on the design of the survey before any irrevocable commitments have been made. Many studies are ruined by failure to take statistical advice at the planning stage.

2. *Data collection.* Consideration should be given to how the data are collected and by whom. Sometimes, skilled interviewers are used and they may require some training prior to being sent out on their assignments.

3. *Questionnaires.* These will be considered in detail later. Many satisfaction surveys have used the questionnaire method. Decisions will have to be made on their format, length and type of question. Bear in mind that an initial exploration of the literature may reveal a questionnaire which has been validated and used elsewhere and will serve the present purpose.

4. *Errors and bias.* Such errors as miscoding can occur and steps may have to be taken to reduce such occurrences. The work of coding clerks can be checked but this raises questions of time and monetary costs. Bias can also occur. For instance, sampling from a telephone directory to obtain the views of the public can be biased, as a proportion of the population do not have telephones and their views may be different from those sampled.

5. *Data handling and processing.* Consideration must be given to how the data obtained will be processed and analysed. It may be necessary to design the forms so that they can be easily coded for computer use, and the necessary software packages for storing the data on computer and for their analysis may have to be obtained.

6. *Identification of resources required.* The number of staff required will have to be identified and funds for materials obtained.

7. *Timing.* Decisions will have to be made as to when to start and when to finish the survey. Normally it is important not to conduct the survey at unrepresentative times, e.g. over the Christmas holidays.

8. *Pilot surveys.* It is good practice to conduct a pilot survey so that errors in the design of questionnaires or difficulties for interviewers can be determined and corrected. During this phase of the investigation, it may be noted that some of the people interviewed are misunderstanding a question and therefore the question needs amending before the definitive study. Another common problem is the language used. A questionnaire may be incomprehensible to the group being investigated. The wording, therefore, needs to be simplified and technical terms avoided. Though the pilot survey will usually identify some problems, snags can still occur in the definitive survey due to the complexity of conducting a bigger operation. The pilot, however, has another use. It gives the person responsible for the proposed survey an opportunity to review whether in the light of what has occurred and what has been found in the pilot survey, it is still worthwhile conducting the main survey. In other words, the pilot survey is a safeguard against the possibility that the main survey may be ineffective.

Many of the technical issues mentioned above apply to any kind of study. They are discussed in more detail in Chapter 11.

Questionnaires

Questionnaires should be differentiated from *recording schedules*. A recording schedule is used by an interviewer who asks the question and records the answer, whereas a questionnaire is filled in by the respondent. The set-up and style of a questionnaire will usually differ from that of a recording schedule. The latter document is designed for efficient field handling and attractiveness may not be part of the design. In contrast, the attractiveness of the questionnaire is often very important as it can lead to higher response ratios. Attention has to be paid to how the questions are set out and clear understandable instructions incorporated such as to show whether certain questions should be answered by only a subset of the population under study. The tools the designer of a questionnaire uses are historical precedents obtained from a literature search, knowledge of the population to be surveyed and of the topic, common sense, past experience and knowledge gained from the pilot survey. A temptation which must be resisted is to make the questionnaire too long. Long questionnaires are likely to increase the refusal rate and affect the quality of the data. Designers of questionnaires should constantly be asking themselves, what will I gain by adding this question?

Question content

People's ability must be taken into account when considering the content of the questions. The questions should be ones that the respondent could be expected to answer accurately. If one is enquiring about past events (e.g. a stay in hospital), then the person consulted might reasonably be expected to have remembered them accurately especially if prompted. If, for instance, one was interested in the attitudes of senile demented patients to a recent hospital admission, then the above conditions will be unlikely to have been met. Also, a person's opinions should be sought only if one is fairly sure that the questions are understandable and the respondent can give meaningful answers. Social conditioning can affect the respondent's reply; for example, women sometimes deliberately underestimate their age and men may inflate their occupational status.

There are three broad types of questions: factual ones, those dealing with opinion, and those dealing with motivation. Classification questions such as date of birth and marital status, which are a special group of factual questions, are often asked at the end of the questionnaire. More confidence is usually placed in factual questions than in opinion questions. This is because a person's opinion on an issue is often not black or white but grey. Depending on the issue, a person may feel very intensely about it or not at all. People's opinions often vary over time and opinion questions are very sensitive to changes in wording and emphasis. Similar considerations apply to motivation questions.

Open vs *closed questions*

An open question does not presuppose the range of responses an individual may give, whereas a closed question does. For example, in a study of out-patient attenders, one may ask 'What improvements should be made to this service?'; this is an open question and the range of response is solely dependent upon the imagination of the patients. In closed form, the question could be put as:

Which of the following aspects of the out-patient service need improvement?

Ambulance services to the clinic
Waiting times in the clinic
Refreshment facilities
Seating arrangements
Information given by doctors, etc.

The closed form presupposes the responses of interest to the investigator, which may not be matters of greatest importance to the patient, and allows for no other possibilities unless a catch-all option is added such as 'Other – please state'. There is no doubt that closed questions are much easier to deal with analytically. However, the best of both worlds may be obtained if a questionnaire is piloted with open questions, the responses to which are used to aid the design of closed questions for a subsequent questionnaire (this should also be piloted).

A questionnaire may have a mixture of both kinds of question. In general, open questions are best asked by an interviewer who has been given explicit instructions as to how far he or she should prompt people's memories and encourage responses.

Wording of questions

There are a number of points to be considered. Simplicity of language has already been alluded to and there are computer programs which will highlight words which are inappropriate for specific age groups. For instance, if one were interested in the attitudes of patients aged 5–8 years to the nurses in a children's ward, then it would be necessary to couch the interview at the appropriate language level.

Other problems that can arise is that the question can be ambiguous or too general. Leading questions on the lines of 'should not something be done about . . .' should in general be avoided. Hypothetical questions such as 'would you like a million pounds' in general contribute little of value. It is only if the person has experience of that state that the opinion becomes of more interest.

Layout of questionnaires

The layout of self-administered questionnaires is as important as the content. The textual characters should be of adequate size for most people's vision, the form should not be overcrowded with text and should run to no more than a couple of pages. Leave sufficient space for people with above-average sized handwriting to mark their responses. It is a useful ploy to leave a large space at the end for 'further comments'; this helps prevent people writing irrelevant remarks on the main body of the questionnaire. Ideally, questionnaires should be professionally printed, because people respond better to a quality product than to an amateurish one; however, if this is beyond the budget, ensure that good-quality office reproduction is used – laser printers are a great boon.

Interviews

Besides self-reporting questionnaires, patient or client satisfaction with a service can be elicited by interviews. Much depends on the skill and training of the interviewer. The characteristics of a good interviewer are honesty and an interest in the subject matter under investigation. In addition, the person should be dependable in that he or she accurately records the information obtained. The personality and temperament of the interviewer are of the utmost importance – good rapport must be established with the person being interviewed. While high degrees of intelligence are not necessary, the interviewer must be able to comprehend instructions.

Training of interviewers

Sometimes this is done by assigning newly appointed staff to already well-trained personnel so that they can accompany them and watch how they conduct their interviews. In other words, on-the-job training is one possibility. Another is a formal training course where the new member of staff conducts mock interviews and these are then criticized. The cheapest method is to supply the new interviewer with written instructions on how to conduct the interview.

Conducting interviews

Obtaining access to the person to be interviewed can be difficult. A prior communication asking if it is permissible to call at a specific time is often helpful. Such letters should be drafted with care and tell the person being interviewed why your organization wishes to encroach on their time. The interviewer should have some credentials that can be shown to the interviewee before the interview begins. Attention should also be given to how the interviewers introduce themselves. An interviewer may say 'My name is Alan Jones and I am employed by your local health authority to get your views on our local service. All answers will be treated in strict confidence.' Once rapport has been established, the interviewer can then proceed to ask the questions. One is aiming for uniformity in approach and recording between interviewers.

Opinion questions are more sensitive than factual questions to variations in wording or voice, and therefore it is very important that interviewers are trained to use uniform wording. Undue emphasis on particular words should also be avoided.

One of the most difficult tasks of the interviewer is to assess the adequacy of the response. One type of inadequate response is the partial response, i.e. the interviewee gives a relevant but incomplete response. The interviewer should avoid the trap of asking a supplementary question on the spur of the moment. It is difficult to form a neutral unbiased supplementary question at short notice. Encouragement might be given by allowing a brief expectant pause to develop.

Other types of inadequate response include non-responses, when the respondent does not answer the question, and irrelevant responses, where the respondent fails to answer the question asked. Inaccurate responses also cause a problem; the interviewee in this case gives a distorted or biased reply to the question asked. Respondent's may also state that they do not understand the question or do not have the knowledge necessary to answer the question. The skill of the interviewer lies in handling inadequate response problems and encouragement might be given by using phrases such as 'I see' or 'Uh-huh'. Surveyors' handbooks often contain specific phrases which can be used for probing for more information.

Postal surveys

Postal surveys, in theory, allow a large number of potential respondents to be contacted fairly cheaply. However, these tend to elicit a low response. Multiple mail-shots to non-respondents usually increase the overall yield.

Some examples

Reid and McIlwaine[2] looked at consumer opinion of a hospital antenatal clinic. An interview schedule was devised which contained both open and closed questions and after a pilot run the questionnaire was administered by a social scientist. A good response ratio was obtained (96%). On analysis, it was found that consumers had three main areas of concern. First were practical considerations relating to clinic visits, e.g. where to place their children while they attended. Also, some patients felt that they received an inadequate explanation from the doctor and from what was taught and explained at the antenatal classes. Deficiencies in mothercraft teaching were identified.

In 1983, the Community Health Council of Burnley, Pendle and Rossendale participated in a survey report[3] of public opinion on the health services of Barnoldswick, an area within the Burnley Health District. A random sample of 12.5% of the electorate was drawn from the Register of Electors, the sample size being approximately 1000. There was a low response ratio (43.3%) despite the active participation of both the community health council and of volunteers from the neighbourhood council. This illustrates the difficulty in getting a good response. Of those who replied, some were dissatisfied with the reception facilities of their GP. A recommendation was made that reception staff should be reoriented in the skills of dealing with often overwrought patients and relatives.

Ann Cartwright and Robert Anderson[4] reported on patients' views and criticisms of GP care. Some of their results are summarized in Table 8.1. These results can be interpreted as either GP services having deteriorated, or patients having become more critical, or both.

Table 8.1 Percentage change in number of patients critical of aspects of GP service between 1964 and 1967

Aspect	Change (%) (+ = deterioration)
Always visiting when asked	+ 433
Examining people carefully and thoroughly	+ 216
Taking time and not hurrying	+ 233
Listening to what you have to say	+ 233
Explaining things fully	+ 143

Source: Cartwright and Anderson (1981).[4]

With regard to patient satisfaction with hospital care, an extensive study was undertaken by the Kings Fund in 1977.[5] For example, it looked at the hotel functions of hospitals and whether patients received sufficient information. Instructions on how to conduct the survey are available and are informative for anybody who wishes to venture into this field.

In 1984, a study was carried out in Nottingham of patients' expectations of and satisfaction with their nursing care.[6] Data collection was achieved using a structured questionnaire and semistructured interviews with patients. The reliability and validity of the questionnaire was tested. Both content and construct validity (see pp. 147–8) were examined. The questionnaire was submitted to the local ethical committee and approved and informed consent was obtained from each respondent. The questionnaire covered such topics as nurse–patient relationships, e.g. whether the nurse was courteous, whether she explained hospital procedures and ward routines. It also covered the physical environment of the ward and nursing attitudes to visitors and relatives. A number of recommendations for management action resulted from the survey.

In 1987, the North Western Regional Health Authority Operational Survey Section conducted an out-patient survey on patients who had attended out-patient services at the North Manchester General Hospital.[7] The format was that patients received a questionnaire plus a covering letter and they were asked to complete the questionnaire and send it by Freepost in the envelope provided to the operational survey section. The questionnaire used was based on one previously employed in another hospital in the North Western area. This was amended and then piloted before use. In the main trial, 3080 questionnaires were sent out but only 1449 were returned, a response ratio of 47%. The questionnaire covered such matters as how the patient reached the clinic, whether there were any problems on arrival, whether waiting conditions were satisfactory in the out-patient department, what facilities were available while waiting to be seen, how long they had to wait, whether staff were courteous and other matters such as whether it was easy to find the way to other departments. The results were analysed and a number of recommendations made to management (e.g. better signposts). It will be noted that half of those contacted failed to respond. This is an example of one of the problems with postal questionnaires.

A problem with patient satisfaction questionnaires is that they generate a lot of data and this is not easy for managers to handle. At the Bloomsbury Health Authority in 1988, there was an initiative to develop composite patient satisfaction indices based on questionnaires.[8] Managers could then plot the patient satisfaction indices on a month-by-month basis and watch the trends. If satisfaction was dropping, management action would be required. To do this time-trend analysis routinely, a simple automated system needed to be developed. The workers at Bloomsbury have devised simple questionnaires and intend to use optical readers to input data.

How should satisfaction surveys influence management?

Finally, there is the question of the weight managers should place on public or patients' perceptions. It is obviously a matter of judgement, but the problem is illustrated in the following example taken from a survey conducted by Southern Sheffield Community Health Council and reported by Trent.[9] Public choices of

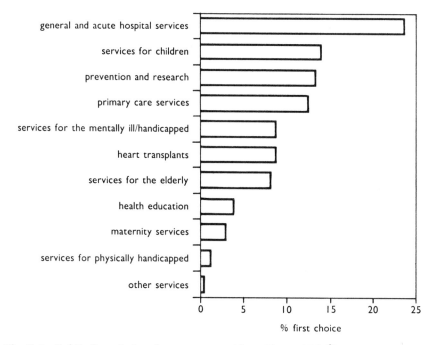

Fig. 8.1   Public first choices for care groups (from Trent, 1981[9]).

priorities for the health service were obtained from a haphazard, but not random, sample of 438 people. The ranking of first choices is displayed in Fig. 8.1. It will be noted that health education does not have a high priority in the public mind, yet many health professionals would argue that major improvements in the health of the population can be obtained through health education programmes, i.e. this is an example of a dichotomy between professional and lay views which managers have to resolve on the basis of their beliefs (see Chapter 12).

Chapter 9

The evaluation of disease prevention services

Introduction

Disease prevention can be classified as primary prevention, secondary prevention or tertiary prevention. The objective of a *primary* prevention programme is to prevent the onset of a disease. An immunization programme, such as that against poliomyelitis, is an example of primary prevention: its objective is to prevent the disease poliomyelitis occurring and its success or failure can be evaluated by noting the number of cases of poliomyelitis which arise in the community. More difficult to evaluate are those primary prevention programmes aimed at reducing risk factors for a disease such as coronary heart disease. Such programmes can be very expensive and therefore their cost-effectiveness needs to be considered. An example of a successful outcome is given later in this chapter.

Secondary prevention is concerned with the early detection of a disease; the assumption being that if the disease is detected earlier, therapy will be more effective. Screening for breast cancer is an example of a secondary prevention programme and this will be discussed in more detail later in this chapter. Finally, the aim of *tertiary* prevention is to slow the progress of established disease or improve the quality of life remaining for such patients.

Health promotion, which has been defined as 'any combination of health education and related organisational, economic and environmental supports for behaviour of individuals, groups or communities conducive to health'[1] can span the three subdivisions of prevention. Many health promotion activities assume there is a linked chain of events thus:

Poor health because of poor knowledge of health risks

Knowledge (e.g. about how to reduce a health risk)

Attitudes (e.g. wanting to reduce that health risk)

Behaviour (e.g. reducing that health risk)

Improved health

For instance, a mass media programme raising community awareness to accidents in the home is a primary prevention programme; it would aim to inform, to motivate people to make their houses safe, and to result in people taking appropriate action. The media campaign might be judged successful if the community's level of knowledge of risk factors for home accidents had risen significantly after the campaign.

Setting up cancer support groups is an example of a tertiary prevention health promotion activity; the objective could be to improve the quality of remaining life and evaluation would rest on patients' and their families' satisfaction with the programme.

Managers work within fixed resources and are therefore (unless they are very fortunate) faced with choices. One common choice is whether to spend a certain amount of resource on prevention or on curative services. To make an informed choice, health promotional activities should not be regarded as an act of faith. Projects in this field should be critically scrutinized and appraised. One difficulty is that improvements in health resulting from health promotional activities often become measurable only years or decades later, whereas the time-span for benefits accruing from curative activities is much shorter. For this reason, evaluation is often in terms of showing that the population at risk has a better knowledge of the disease and of risk factors, and that attitudes and behaviour have changed. Moreover, scientifically credible and statistically robust studies frequently have to be on a large scale – most districts cannot undertake these and so evidence of a health promotion project's likelihood of success usually rests on results from national or international studies. Such studies should be quoted in the application for funding.

The North Karelia study: An example of the evaluation of primary prevention

An example of a national study which had an impact on local health promotion is some work which took place in Finland in the 1970s. At that time, Finland had a very high rate of coronary heart disease. A project was set up in one of the Finnish provinces, North Karelia, with the following aims:

- to reduce risk factors for coronary heart disease such as the prevalence of smoking, high blood pressure or high serum cholesterol;
- to decrease morbidity and mortality from coronary heart disease; and
- to detect, treat and follow-up patients with high blood pressure.

A baseline survey was conducted prior to the intervention. A total of 11,500 people were asked to participate, and a 90% response was achieved. The baseline survey was followed by five follow-up surveys at 6-monthly intervals each involving a 3.5% random sample of the population. Again, a good response ratio was obtained (82–91%).

The intervention was started in 1972 and consisted of giving the public information through public meetings and media coverage; for instance, attention was drawn to the sale of low-fat milk and low-fat sausages. Doctors were involved in the project because of their role as key health professionals. Training was given to a variety of other health professionals. The findings from the study were published[2,3] in 1979 and some of them are shown in Table 9.1.

Table 9.1   Some results from the North Karelia study

	Baselines (%)	Last follow-up (%)	Difference (%)
Smokers			
men	54	42	− 12
women	12	12	0
Use of butter	86	72	− 14
Use of low-fat milk	17	41	+ 24
Blood pressure measured in last 3 months	28	56	+ 28

The success of the project can be judged by the lowering of risk factors and by increased population awareness. In Wales, coronary artery disease rates are also high and the evidence quoted above helped to make the case for government support for a similar project to the North Karelia project called Heartbeat Wales.

Managers live in a continually changing environment. Advances in medicine lead to demands for new services and NHS managers are often faced with decisions as to whether to put resources into new techniques or whether to delay implementation. A major factor in such decisions should be a critical analysis of the data. Here, sound medical advice is of the utmost importance, and often the department of public health medicine can offer such assistance. The following examples related to screening illustrate some of the problems at both the national and district levels, and illustrate the importance of a good review of the literature.

Examples of the evaluation of secondary prevention

Breast cancer screening: An expensive medical technique

Breast cancer is a very common form of cancer in women. It has been established that about 15,000 women in the UK die of breast cancer each year. In most parts of the UK, it is the leading cause of female cancer deaths. It is not surprising, therefore, that considerable efforts have been made to reduce mortality from this disease. Screening apparently healthy women for the disease has been one approach adopted. An expensive medical technique (EMT), namely mammography, has been suggested as a breast-screening tool. However, before utilizing EMTs and allocating funds to them, one should be aware of the problems they may produce. We shall develop this theme a little in general terms before returning to the details of breast screening (see also Chapter 10).

Assessing EMTs

There is often a tendency to consider EMTs in isolation and not in competition with other desirable developments or improvements. Also, one is often faced with what has been called the technological imperative, i.e. to take action whatever the cost if the EMT offers even the slightest possibility of benefit. Premature jumping on the bandwagon has often in the past produced errors, e.g. the local freezing of stomach ulcers proved ineffective.

Problems with EMTs occur because of public and political pressures generated by often exaggerated claims in the world press. This leads to inadequate evaluation before their introduction. Another problem is that they may lead to specialist units for a minority which results in resources being taken away from the majority. It should be noted that the revenue consequences of EMTs are often very high, since specialized manpower is required. Special-care baby units are a good example of this and the inappropriate use of such facilities can escalate costs. Moreover, many EMTs make diagnosis more precise or earlier. However, it is often uncertain if their use reduces mortality or morbidity.

Managers should ask whether an EMT is efficacious, reliable, effective and whether it is able to distinguish between diseased and normal. Managers need also to consider the full costs of an EMT. These include:

1. Capital costs (write-off time).
2. Space requirements (alterations or buildings needed).
3. Revenue costs under the following headings:
   - staff,
   - consumables,
   - maintenance, and
   - additional energy and transport costs.
4. Effect on patient services and knock-on effects.

Finally, the key question is not whether an EMT is beneficial but whether it is beneficial enough to deserve a high priority, and that question should be answered in the affirmative before proceeding. A checklist to aid in these decisions is presented in Appendix B. More details on the evaluation of technology in health care are given in Chapter 10.

Moreover, for any screening programme, certain other specific criteria should be met. Wilson and Jungner[4] formulated the following principles of screening for the World Health Organization and these are cited in the Forrest Report[9] (see below):

- the condition sought should pose an important health problem;
- the natural history of the disease should be well understood;
- there should be a recognizable early stage;

- treatment of the disease at an early stage should be of more benefit than treatment started at a later stage;
- there should be a suitable test;
- the test should be acceptable to the population;
- there should be adequate facilities for the diagnosis and treatment of abnormalities detected;
- for diseases of insidious onset, screening should be repeated at intervals determined by the natural history of the disease;
- the chance of physical or psychological harm to those screened should be less than the chance of benefit;
- the cost of a screening programme should be balanced against the benefit it provides.

Is breast cancer screening worthwhile?

Several reasons have been advanced for routine mass breast screening. One reason is that earlier diagnosis leads to better survival. The argument goes that large tumours are more likely to have metastasized to local lymph glands or distant sites than small tumours. Breast cancer may be detected *in situ* before they have become invasive. This assumes that in the natural history of the disease, tumour size correlates with metastatic spread and this may not be true especially for blood-borne spread. Another reason is that screening followed by appropriate action can lead to a reduction in mortality.

In 1985, the Department of Health was interested in the possibility of breast screening. Evidence in favour came from the New York (HIP) study[5] and two Dutch studies, one from Nijmegen[6] and one from Utrecht.[7] In March 1985, the Department of Health received a pre-publication copy of the Swedish two-countries study,[8] which also came out in favour of mammographic screening. In view of this, the department was able to advise the then minisiter that the moment had come to reappraise policy. He announced the setting up of the Forrest Committee to advise the government on the issue of breast-screening on the same day as the Swedish paper was published in the *Lancet*, namely 13 April 1985. As a result of the Forrest Report,[9] a national breast-screening programme was initiated. It should be stated that the government *pre-empted* the randomized clinical trial conducted in the UK.[10] The findings from these studies are summarized in Table 9.2.

Breast screening is now national policy in the UK. There is some evidence that it may have been introduced prematurely. Recent clinical trials (e.g. the Edinburgh study[10]: see Table 9.2) failed to show that mammographic screening lowered the mortality rate by a statistically significant amount. Such studies have been challenged by those in favour of screening on grounds such as an inadequate coverage of the population. Knock-on effects of the EMT are beginning to show, surgeons are complaining they are unable to cope with the demand and their waiting lists are rising. As a case study, the implementation of mammography is interesting because it shows the disadvantages of taking a decision before all the evidence is in. It was known that the major UK trial was

Table 9.2   Breast cancer screening studies which have reported an effect on mortality

Place	Design	Screening method	Age group (years)	Interval (years)	Reduction in mortality (%)
HIP	RCT[a]	Clinical + 2-view mammography	40–64	1	30 New York
Sweden	RCT	1-view mammography	40 and over	1.5–3	31
Nijmegen	Case, control	1-view mammography	35 and over	2	52
Utrecht	Case, control	Clinical + 2-view mammography	50–64	1–4	70
Florence	Case, control	2-view mammography	40–70	2.5	50
Edinburgh	RCT	Clinical + mammography: 2-view initially, 1-view on follow-up	45–64	2	17[b]

Additional sources not already referenced in text: Day *et al* (1986)[11] and Baines (1987).[12]
[a] Randomized controlled trial
[b] Not statistically significant.

Table 9.3   A comparison of event rates for certain conditions as reported from six trials on the treatment of mild hypertension

	Trial[a]					
	VACS	USPHS	ANBPS	OSLO	MRC	EWHPE
Non-fatal strokes	+	+	+[b]	+	+	+
Deaths, all causes	+	+	+	−	+	+
Deaths, cardiovascular	+	+	+[b]	−	+	+[b]
Deaths, cardiac	+	+	+	−	−	+[b]
Deaths, stroke	+	None	+	+	+	+
All strokes: fatal plus non-fatal	+	+	+[b]	+[b]	+[b]	+

[a] VACS, Veterans Administration Cooperative study;[13] USPHS, US Public Hospitals Service Cooperative Study;[14] ANBPS, Australian trial;[15] OSLO, Oslo Study;[16] MRC, Medical Research Council study;[17] EWHPE, European Working Party on high blood pressure in the elderly study.[18]
[b] Significant at the P<0.05 level.
Sample difference: + = the event rate was lower in the treatment group; − = the event rate was lower in the control group.

in progress when the political decision was taken and sufficient account does not appear to have been taken of the knock-on effects of breast screening on other services such as surgery.

Screening for mild hypertension

By the beginning of the 1960s, there was considerable evidence that treatment of moderate or severe hypertension was of benefit to patients with cardio-vascular disease. The question beginning to exercise people's minds was whether there was any merit in treating patients with mild hypertension and, if there was, whether a screening programme should be initiated.

A critical analysis of clinical trials could answer the first question. Table 9.3 lists six trials. First, note that as far as cardiac deaths are concerned, two trials failed to show any benefit from treatment and one of these was the Medical Research Council (MRC) large-scale trial in the UK. Secondly, note that all trials showed that treatment was of benefit in regard to reducing the incidence of strokes (fatal and non-fatal).

Table 9.4 illustrates an important point that needs to be considered, namely statistical analysis. In one trial, statistical significance was not calculated; two others did not state whether differences between treated and controls achieved statistical significance. One is likely therefore to attach less weight to such trials.

It is important to know not only that treatment reduces strokes, and that this reduction is not a statistical artefact, but also the magnitude of that benefit. This can be calculated and was undertaken for three trials (Table 9.5). It will

Table 9.4 Comparison of findings from six trials on the treatment of mild hypertension[a,b]

Trial	Treatment group	Control group	Is the rate lower in the treatment group?	Does the difference achieve statistical significance?
VACS	8.4	31.2	Yes	Unstated
USPHS	0.7	4.4	Yes	Unstated
ANBPS	2.4	4.5	Yes	Yes ($P<0.025$)
OSLO	0	3.4	Yes	Yes ($P<0.02$)
MRC	1.4	2.6	Yes	Yes ($P<0.01$ on sequential analysis)
EWHPE	23	38	Yes	Not calculated

[a] The outcome under consideration is all strokes (fatal and non-fatal) measured as rates per 1000 subject years of treatment.
[b] See Table 9.3 for key and references.

Table 9.5 Calculated 95% confidence intervals for the absolute difference in total stroke per 1000 subject years of treatment

Trial	95% confidence interval
ANBPS	0.1–4.1
OSLO	0.9–5.9
MRC	0.6–1.7

See Table 9.3 for key and references.

be noted that the 95% confidence limit of the MRC trial embraces a narrower range and this is due to the larger size of this trial as compared to the other two. Using this as a basis, it can be seen that benefit per 1000 years of treatment is relatively small.

Before embarking on a screening programme, the criteria mentioned earlier for screening should be considered. Screening for hypertension can produce harm: being labelled hypertensive has consequences, e.g. higher insurance premiums, and drugs used for treatment can have harmful effects. These effects must be weighed against benefit. The cost-utility (see pp. 68–75) should also be borne in mind. The estimated cost per quality-adjusted life year for screening for hypertension has been estimated as £1700, compared to £3000–5000 per quality-adjusted life year for breast screening. (For reservations about the use of quality-adjusted life years, see p. 71).

Opportunity costs should also be considered. Table 9.6 shows some data from the MRC trial. It can be seen that for strokes (and it was also shown for all cardio-vascular events), the difference between the rates in smokers and non-smokers was greater than the difference between treatment and control groups. Additionally, this simple finding demonstrates a lower stroke rate in the non-smokers on placebo medication than in the smokers who took routine hypotensive agents. These results from the MRC trial therefore suggest that it is probably more important that subjects refrain from smoking than have their mildly raised blood pressure treated.

It could thus be argued that if district resources are limited, the first priority for districts wishing to reduce strokes is to reduce smoking in their population

Table 9.6 Impact of smoking on outcome in the MRC trial of treatment for mild hypertension

Strokes per 1000 subject years (intention to treat analysis)	Smokers	Non-smokers
Treatment group	2.6	0.9
Control group	3.9	2.0

See table 9.3 for key and references.

rather than embarking on screening their population for hypertension, especially as the screening cost per quality-adjusted life year for smoking is estimated to be £180.

In summary, a critical evaluation of clinical trials can help determine policy. Failure to take this step can result in an unwise use of resources.

Evaluating tertiary prevention

Examples have been given of trials in primary and secondary prevention. Trials in tertiary prevention are often difficult to perform due to a number of confounding factors. For instance, trials to ascertain whether rehabilitation is of value in stroke have been carried out, but one must be aware when interpreting the results that it is difficult to match 'control' and 'trial' subjects, the extent of the stroke can differ and in addition such people often have other pathology.

Garraway *et al*[19] compared the management of elderly patients with acute stroke, randomized either to a stroke unit or to a medical ward. A better short-term outcome (mean of 60 days) was noted and the difference was statistically significant ($P<0.001$). It was noted that stroke physiotherapy was given markedly earlier and that the duration of treatment and number of hours of treatment were clearly less than those given on the medical units. On the basis of these results, and from a manager's point of view, early short-term physiotherapy is required. It is interesting to note that in the follow-up study[20] differences in functional outcome had disappeared after 1 year. This emphasizes the importance of looking at long-term outcomes as well as short-term outcomes.

Sivenius *et al*[21] carried out a control trial on stroke. They compared the effectiveness of two intensities of physiotherapy and found that functional recovery after stroke as measured by activities of daily living and motor function was markedly better in the intensified therapy group, i.e. the main gain being in the first 3 months.

Chapter 10

Technology assessment

Introduction

It has been eloquently argued by Donabedian[1] that although at first sight the evaluation of technology and the assessment of quality appear very different, it is impossible to isolate one from the other. We sympathize with this view, but feel that, none the less, special consideration needs to be given to some particular features of the evaluation of health care technology. The impact of health care technologies on quality can happen in a number of ways: they can reduce the costs of achieving a given benefit, or open the way to achieving benefits hitherto thought impossible. As has been argued previously about evaluating health services generally, the evaluation of technology should theoretically only be undertaken if one is aware of the full range of potential implications – financial, social, behavioural and biological. By this we mean that the costs should always be recognized; that the benefits may have enormous implications for society as well as the individual; that the use and evaluation of a technology is governed by attitudes towards it; and that its contribution in purely biological terms is but one facet of a complex interplay of all these factors.

Before we progress further, a working definition of 'technology' is required. Readers will find that the technology assessment literature covers a huge range of topics, from the visibly very 'high-tech', such as magnetic resonance imaging, through the medium-technology of diagnostic procedures such as gastroscopy or echocardiography, to the relatively low-technology of urine screening, vaccines and cervical smears. Some of the characteristics of types of technology are summarized in Table 10.1. It can be seen that they are largely the *instruments* of care, i.e. the tools of the trade. Schon[2] provides a useful definition: 'Any tool or technique, any physical equipment or method of doing or making, by which human capability is extended.'

There are five characteristics to be considered when looking at technology: capital investment, size, complexity, user's skills and potential for harm. Note that none of these has a direct relationship with health benefits. Definitions of

Table 10.1   Characteristics of different kinds of medical technology

Characteristic	Types of technology		
	High-technology	Medium-technology	Low-technology
Initial capital investment	Very high (can run to millions of pounds)	Medium (up to £50,000)	Very low (at times only a few pence)
Size	Large	Medium	Small
Complexity	Very high	Moderate	Apparently low
Required skills of users	Wide range (high for using the machine: MRI; high for interpreting results: CT)	Wide range (invasive techniques require high skills; imaging requires high interpreting skills)	Apparently very low (but inappropriately taken cervical smears are no use)
Potential for harm to the individual patient	High from therapeutic technology, such as radiotherapy; otherwise potentially very little	High for many invasive technologies	Generally extremely low to the individual, but appreciable over populations
Main users	Apart from radiotherapy, usually diagnostic specialities	A mixture of diagnostic and therapeutic specialities; includes organ transplant	Dominated by preventive specialities, as well as therapeutic and diagnostic technologies
Market size	Generally very small	Moderate	Whole populations

high- and medium-technology usually imply a direct relationship with capital investment, size and complexity. Thus there is no doubt that radiotherapeutic technology and diagnostic technology are 'high-tech': the machines occupy whole rooms, cost vast sums, and work only because of an incredibly imaginative harnessing of computerized detail to an understanding and vision of human anatomy and physiology. Sometimes this complexity demands a complementary high skill from users, as in radiotherapy and magnetic resonance imaging (MRI); sometimes, however, the skill is not so much in the use of the machine as in interpreting what it reveals, e.g. this applies in particular to computerized tomography (CT).

As a result, it would be tempting to disregard low-technology; it is generally cheaper, requires less skill and is less liable to be damaging to the individual. But because of these characteristics, low-technology is more likely to be taken up on a massive scale and to be applied for the benefit of millions of people, whole populations, and not just for a few hundreds as with high-technology, or even thousands as with medium-technology. The result is that the total cost of a low-technology, in both financial and human terms, may be greater than any high-technology instrument; there is also potential for enormous population benefits.

Every form of technology merits evaluation; none should be ignored. The process of evaluation will involve all that we have already covered in preceding chapters. There are, however, three special features which need particularly careful consideration and these will now be discussed in more detail: costs, underlying ideologies and statistical considerations.

Costs

General accounting and economic considerations pertinent to evaluation have been considered in Chapter 5. There are six types of cost which require emphasis in any evaluation of technology and health care: capital costs, maintenance, running costs, training costs, replacement costs and service implication costs. They are largely *accounting* costs. However, there are related *economic* concepts which will be brought out.

Capital costs

Capital costs are the size of the initial investment in a technology. They can be substantial; millions of pounds may have to be spent to acquire radio-therapeutic equipment. As such, they represent a very high proportion of the fixed costs of a service, as a one-off spend; for low-technology services, the capital costs can be minimal – perhaps just a couch and a light for taking cervical smears.

The capital investment has one major and visible characteristic: it is non-consumable, and as such remains as an obvious piece of hardware, regardless of the extent to which it is, or is not, used. The NHS is generally criticized for not making the most cost-effective use of its capital. There are, however, other characteristics of a capital investment which, although invisible, are none the less vital as part of any evaluation, let alone as part of any health service manager's recognition of how money has been spent. Prior to the NHS and Community Care Act 1990, the health service was under no obligation to recognize the value of capital investments; the ability to do so is now an essential part of the management job.

The process involves looking at the return on a capital investment. This entails being able to account for the following:

● the initial capital expenditure;
● the rate at which the asset purchased with that expenditure will depreciate;

- how long the asset is likely to be in use, and therefore the period over which depreciation will occur;
- the revenue which could be earned as a result of owning the asset; and
- what else the initial capital investment could have bought, i.e. its opportunity cost.

These are considered in turn below.

The initial capital investment

This is usually straightforward. The purchasing process may be complicated by having to go to tender for expensive items of equipment, although this does have the advantage of requiring a detailed specification to be spelt out, which can be very helpful because it should define the objectives of the technology. Complicating issues arise if the equipment is purchased from abroad, as there will be considerations affecting exchange rates and there may also be regulations governing the use of intellectual property. Equipment purchased for research may be exempt of value-added tax. Particularly large items of equipment may incur a cost not only for the equipment but also for its accommodation; air conditioning, X-ray (lead) screening or other specialist designed features may be needed. This will not only add to the cost of the effort, but also influence the time-scale over which the money is spent.

Depreciation

Every car owner (apart from the exceptional few who own vintage vehicles) knows that cars depreciate in value over time. It is also generally recognized that some cars lose a high proportion of their value at a very early age, and then retain a fairly constant value, whereas others lose value at a slower and steadier rate. The same applies to a health technology capital asset. It is tempting to assume that such an asset will lose value at a steady rate over a given time, such as 10 years, because the accounting calculations are so much simpler in this *straight line* depreciation. But it may be quite unrelated to what really happens. Many major items of medical equipment may retain their value to a high proportion of the initial investment for the first 3–4 years of the technology's life; thereafter, the value may drop precipitately. Each type of equipment has a characteristic pattern of depreciation, and it is highly desirable to use this, and not oversimple assumptions, if good-quality accounting or evaluation are to be practised.

Lifetime

The life of any given type of health care technology can be very difficult to estimate. Conventionally, 8–10 years is the time-span used. We all know of equipment which has been kept functioning way beyond that, and also of equipment which has been redundant almost as soon as it is purchased because it has been superseded by a newer, better technology. None the less, an estimate or even 'guesstimate' is necessary, because it underpins so many of the other aspects of measuring the return on capital investment. When the initial investment has been very high, it may be worth spending money to canvass expert opinion locally, nationally and even internationally, to arrive at as well-informed an opinion as possible.

Revenue earned

Prior to the NHS and Community Care Act 1990, any health care technology would only be costed in terms of the expenditure required to use it; now it is necessary to ensure that all health services are paid for. The assessment of revenue earned by a health care technology will include knowledge of whether or not it appears to meet a well-recognized and priority health need (i.e. what the NHS market is for the technology), whether potential purchasers are likely to receive development funds (based on national assumptions and local resource allocation procedures), and whether there is a private sector demand. The price to be charged would relate to all of these, to the fixed and variable costs of the technology, and to the type of contract regarding its use.

The opportunity cost

In the private sector, and probably increasingly in the NHS, this will involve two main decisions:

● what other technology the money could have been spent on, and what that technology could have earned; and
● how else the money could have been invested, and what that would have earned.

The first question would have been anticipated and will, no doubt, have been an integral part of the discussions leading to a decision to purchase a technology after evaluation. The second is especially relevant to the business sector where, for example, over 10 years of an asset's lifetime, it may earn a great deal more, or less, than if the money had simply been invested in, say, government bonds. The calculation involves discounting (as defined in Chapter 5), and provides a summary figure covering the relevant time-scale: the *net present value* (any management accounting text will give details). The value of calculating a net present value, and hence the return on the capital investment, is that it makes the opportunity cost of an investment quite explicit, and demonstrates that organizations have to think very carefully about their objectives in investing in a given technology, in order to judge whether or not such an investment really is worthwhile.

Maintenance costs

Maintenance costs should be relatively straightforward to estimate, and will in any case be quantified in any substantial purchase of an expensive technology for which a detailed specification has been written. These costs are really part of a running cost of any technology but are identified separately because the price of a technology may include in the maintenance agreement important aspects like the availability of a 24-hour repair service, free replacements of parts within a given time-scale, and the willingness of the manufacturer to service the equipment at unsocial hours so that it is their technicians, and not the hospital staff or patients, who are inconvenienced.

Running costs

The revenue implications of a health care technology are no trivial matter, as any manager knows. All too often in the past, charities raised funds for expensive equipment, only to find that the would-be benefactor could not afford to accept their gift. Revenue implications include the maintenance of equipment, and also the consumables required to make it usable: X-ray films, laboratory reagents and the like. There will be staff costs, and if the equipment can only be used by highly skilled and rare personnel, these may be considerable. NHS Trusts may, if they are offering salaries and terms and conditions of service which differ from those in the NHS generally, find it difficult to estimate staff costs. There will also be accommodation costs: heat, light, power and maintaining the required environment. Even low-technology like vaccines have running costs: refrigeration, stock control, syringes and needles, an environment in which they can be given, and staff to do the work. As NHS accounting becomes more sophisticated and detailed, so it will be increasingly feasible to allocate an institution's revenue appropriately to the technologies responsible for those costs. In the meantime, it may only be feasible to look at the marginal impact of an additional technology, i.e. the extra expense likely to be incurred as a result of installing new technology.

Training costs

Training costs, particularly for a new technology, are all too easily forgotten. An example of good practice where training has been costed as part of the investment in a new technology is the NHS Breast Screening Service. It is also exemplary in that specific resources have been set aside for the evaluation of a number of different aspects of the service. The NHS has increasingly recognized that training is required as part of any programme of change; the management training programmes, and the funding for doctors in management introduced as part of the general management function, bear witness to that. As health care becomes more technical, more specialized skills are needed. Training costs will include course fees and expenses, as well as the costs of paying temporary or locum staff to continue the work while the incumbent is away being trained.

Replacement costs

Part of the work required to measure a financial return on investment should include the assessment of replacement costs. The process of *capital charging* is, potentially, a means of forcing the NHS to include replacement costs as part of its accounting procedures. In very general terms, part of the costs of a service (and thus the price charged) will include some sort of reserve which should cover the replacement of the technology. It seems to be a feature of many technologies that the price does not drop over time as one might expect, as manufacturing costs are reduced by economies of scale or scope and increased learning; rather, the prices remain relatively steady, but the 'value-added' increases, such that the performance, sophistication and range of the technology are all enhanced. We are all familiar with this in motor cars; the same holds true for much medical technology. As a result, replacement costs are not simply something which can be left to the accountants. As commented on in respect of the likely life-span of a technology, it may be worth investing resources at an early stage to learn what the increased added-value of future models of the technology will be, and how those changes are likely to affect the service.

Service implication costs

Finally, costs of implications for the service need to be taken into account. An increased ability to diagnose certain diseases using a new technology may lead to an increased desire to offer treatment. This will incur costs. One example relates to the use of ultrasound in pregnancy. It was initially useful for assessing the gestational age of a foetus, largely on the basis of size. With increasing sophistication of both the technology and the staff using it, it is now possible to identify anatomical abnormalities, some of which may be amenable to intra-uterine or early neonatal surgery. A whole new medical technical industry developed as a result, without prior consideration of the costs – both financial and ethical.

Underlying ideologies

The shorter *Oxford English Dictionary* defines ideology as 'the science of ideas; the study of the origin and nature of ideas; ... a system of ideas concerning phenomena, especially those of social life ...'. We have already emphasized the importance of explicating underlying ideologies when undertaking evaluation. Here we describe three of the main ideologies which influence the evaluation of technology and health care. The description is not intended to be exhaustive, but does include concepts which are likely to inform any such evaluation, either wholly or in part. These three ideologies are the product life-cycle concept, organization theory and political science.

Product life-cycle

The *product life-cycle* is a marketing concept. It envisages four periods for any product or technology: product development, an introductory/sales growth period, a maturity period and decline. The types of customer who become involved during the sales growth period have also been characterized: innovators at the very early stage, followed by early adopters, early majority, late majority and laggards. The process is also known as product 'diffusion', which is how much of the literature on this topic is classified. The relationship between 'diffusion' or product sales and time is shown in Fig.10.1. Different patterns imply different types of technology, and it does not seem unreasonable that medical care technologies can also be thought of as 'style', 'fashion' and 'fad'. For example, any theatre sister knows that suture materials, intravenous cannulae and disposable giving sets, enjoy a vogue depending on the preferences of the medical staff using them; these are examples of style. There will always be one type of these technologies in the ascendancy and another in the decline. The 'fashion' curve probably characterizes much technology, where the time spent in the maturity period will depend on whether customers simply replace the technology as it wears out, or if they substitute new technologies for old – in which case the decline will be accelerated. The 'fad' curve may be the way that many non-medical staff conceptualize what seems to them to be unreasonable and remarkably short-lived medical demands for technology. For example, not so long ago, it seemed that every consultant had to have a microcomputer, without realizing the running costs and training costs in terms of their own time; the machines, according to many apocryphal tales, rapidly became neglected dust traps.

How does this approach matter to the evaluation of health service effectiveness? First, there is an invisible but none the less important aspect: the educational role of diffusion or the product life-cycle. The illustrations are purely in terms of financial/quantity of sales terms over time. They imply that eventually the profit or number of products sold would decline to zero. What they cannot show is the learning by the market exposed to the products, even if it does not buy them once, let alone come back for more. Even a short-lived fad has an impact on our communal knowledge, our institutional understanding of a particular type of technology and what can be achieved. Because each technology gives its owner(s) good and bad experiences, there rapidly builds up an informal evaluation and a body of opinion. Greer's[4] study of the relative diffusion of technology in the UK and the USA highlights the importance of informal networks as well as formal evaluations in encouraging a market for medical technologies.

The second reason for using the product life-cycle as an underlying ideology when evaluating health care technology, is that it can play a major role in the type of evaluation taken, and its likely conclusions. It is not difficult to understand that collecting evaluative evidence from 'innovators' will reveal an enthusiasm differing by several orders of magnitude from that of 'laggards'. The pace at which a technology is adopted will influence any evaluation; ultrasound examination in pregnancy has diffused rapidly, and is widely advocated by obstetricians, despite there being little evidence of improved perinatal outcome. How can one evaluate a technology which seems to be in place everywhere?

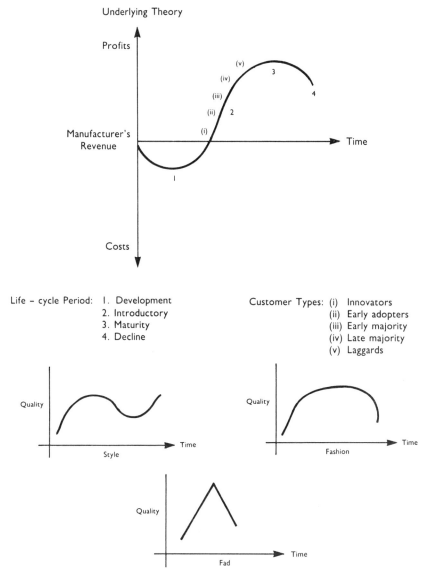

Fig. 10.1 The product life-style

The literature suggests that early adopters change their practice more rapidly than late adopters; in medicine, their behaviour tends to be related to the volume of patients they see for whom the new technology may be useful. The rate of substitution is related to the patient volume, and also, as demonstrated in a recent study by Peddecord *et al.*,[5] shows a 'catch up' phenomenon, because later doctors may substitute more rapidly than innovators, as if making up for lost time.

The conclusion from this is that evaluators must be opportunists when it comes to health care technology, or, as Battista[6] says: '... technologies tend to be diffused before the evaluative studies are completed'. At that stage, the evaluator's ideal of a double-blind case control study is rendered completely impossible.

We suggest that, armed with this insight, managers can take the following action:

1. They can ignore the need for evaluation and assume that the pace of diffusion itself reflects myriad professional evaluations, where only benefit would achieve market success.
2. They can encourage means of learning at an early stage of likely innovations, through formal and informal channels, and send in an evaluative team with the remit to respond in an appropriate time-scale.

The former is consistent with the history of the NHS in it allows local autonomy and provider-driven developments (as described by Harrison).[7] It is also consistent with the ideology underlying the product life-cycle, that for every product there is a market. The idea of *not* using innovations or new technologies is almost unheard of in this approach to life. The second option would require multi-centre collaboration between managers and clinicians in provider units, together with purchasing authorities setting aside funds to evaluate technologies which seem particularly significant. At the time of writing, the structures which would encourage this do not exist. As the impact of health care technologies increasingly complicates decisions about health resource rationing, we feel it is the only way forward.

Organization theory

Evaluators of health care technology may prefer an approach based on organizational theory rather than the product life-cycle, because health care technology only requires evaluation as and when it is desired by the relevant organizations. Here we are using Etzioni's[8] definition of an organization: 'organisations are social units (or human groupings) deliberately constructed and reconstructed to seek specific goals'. The importance of 'goals', and what they mean for a service and for an evaluation, has already been discussed. In Etzioni's definition it implies a common sense of purpose, an agreed direction in life, for the hospital or service. There is a second important component to his definition, i.e. change. He says 'constructed and reconstructed', and this implies a flexibility rather than rigidity, amendment rather than sameness. The evaluator of health care technology may have an ideology relating to an understanding of change in organizations, a management science in its own right.[9-11]

The organizations which impinge on the evaluation of health care technology are included by Donabedian[12] in his description of the structure of health services. Thus they comprise the following:

1. Aspects to do with accessibility: distance, how entrance is gained to a service, its scope, the hours for which it is available.
2. Aspects to do with technical management: physical structure, facilities, equipment, methods of payment, working conditions for staff.
3. Aspects to do with the interpersonnel process: staffing hierarchies, time per patient or procedure, means of obtaining user satisfaction data.

It is not difficult to imagine how the evaluation of a technology from an organizational ideology could find this approach useful. For example, the complex process of evaluating cervical screening, if it is to cover the main features relevant to pragmatic managers, will of necessity have to include the accessibility of the service, the major difficulties encountered in its technical management and the interpersonnel process. The added insight of organization theory comes from recognizing the psychological dynamics of human groupings and, particularly with innovative technology, the impact of change. Thus it is not enough simply to compare the number of cervical smears taken with a given incidence of or mortality rate from cervical cancer. The ideology of organizational theorists allows the systems of health care delivery, and their interaction, to be documented in a manner which can then reveal opportunities for improvement.

Neither the product life-cycle approach nor the organizational theory approach will be perfect for all evaluations of all technologies. Each may use ideas from the other. In addition, they may borrow ideas from political science, and this is explained below.

Political ideologies

Here we define 'political' as: '... of, belonging or pertaining to, the state, its government and policy ... belonging to or taking a side in politics' (shorter *Oxford English Dictionary*). A political ideology can underpin the evaluation of health care technology as much as it can underlie any evaluation. There are three main political influences on the evaluation of health care technology. They are the relative power of medical specialities, issues of control and the process of change. These are discussed in turn below.

Relative medical power

The main impact of medical power may be whether or not a technology is ever evaluated. The stereotype of the medical power dichotomy must be the hospital consultant *vs* the community health/preventive doctor. We would argue that where the power is greater, the ability to evaluate is proportionally diminished, because it is impossible for anyone to entertain a disinterested point of view. Examples of this are the impossibility of evaluating lithotripsy in this country[13] and, more recently, the paucity of evaluation of magnetic resonance imaging (MRI), as noted in the paper by Peddecord and colleagues.[5] With respect to MRI, the Department of Health commissioned a meeting from which health authorities could take advice about whether or not to commission this technology; the conclusions of the meeting were published but not in a peer reviewed journal; nevertheless this form of publication was sufficient for the conclusions to be studied and debated. As Battista[6] says:

> Companies developing high technologies often operate like oligopolies or monopolies. This explains ... the high prices ... [and] ... the obsolescence of expensive equipment ... in general ... the technologies tend to be diffused before the evaluative studies are completed.

The political power structure is probably also reinforced by what is known as 'anticipated decision regret', i.e. the imperative nature of medical technology, particularly high-technology, which applies as a phenomenon to the medical profession and to patients.[14] Again, this can make evaluation virtually impossible, or extremely difficult to complete.

By contrast, relatively low-technologies are not seen as worth taking a risk for. Vaccination against whooping cough is a prime example. Work continues to develop a vaccine that is less reactogenic and more immunogenic than current whole-cell vaccines; an acellular preparation is available and is now subject to stringent trials (for example, see Miller *et al.*).[15] This is as it should be. It is tempting to conclude, however, that requirements for demonstrable safety and efficacy are markedly different for the different technologies.

Issues of control

Here the situation is reversed, in the UK anyway. Although there is generally no central policy regarding technical innovations, and little insistence on the demonstration of clinical efficacy rather than technical safety, at this stage the central financing system enables a limit to be placed on overall spending, and medical technologies compete for funding within allocated budgets. It is of course impossible to predict if this will change, but currently there is very tight control exercised on the diffusion of very expensive high-technology. The control is unrelated to health needs; it is a financial imperative dictated to the service politically by the cash-limited funding allocated to health authorities by parliamentary vote. The cheaper the technology, the less it is controlled, as far as its purchase is concerned. There are of course rules in this game.[16] There are virtually always some non-recurrent underspendings at the end of the financial year, which can be awarded at the discretion of authority officers, and they are highly likely to share the same priorities and sensitivity to medical power as their clinical colleagues, so that in the end the more powerful specialities are likely to win again. We would hope that in future the emphasis on being able to relate services (and their technologies) to population health needs will encourage a more discriminatory and expert control in which evaluation plays an integral part.

Politics and change

This is, again, only mentioned so that would-be evaluators, or commissioners of evaluations, are aware that their approach and ideas regarding the evaluation of a technology may be influenced by local politics and local change. No one can be completely distanced from the real life of the service, or they would not care about evaluation anyway. Politically, an organization can undergo several types of change, of which repetitive, adaptive and radical are the most readily characterized.[16] In *repetitive* change, political structures cope with disturbances in the environment without changing their form. They have rules which ensure that equilibrium is restored. The retirement of senior consultants is an example; local 'rules' are highly likely to be effective in ensuring that the chosen successor does not disturb the established power structure. The naïve evaluator may hope that the appointment of an energetic young consultant will permit all sorts of evaluation and challenges to be mounted which were hitherto unthinkable. Unfortunately (and we speak from experience), this is often not the case: Unless, of course, the political structure sees an advantage in adjustments, and so changes the rules. This is adaptive change and, if the evaluator is sensitive to it, provides an excellent opportunity. It necessitates a rapid response and a willingness to drop other work to pick up something new. The pay-off is that as a new structure settles and ensures that the local rules now perpetuate its new equilibrium, so evaluation – and the evaluation team – will be incorporated into the new structure.

Further opportunity, in theory at least, is available at times of *radical* change, but the changes may be so dramatic and so complete that it is impossible to define an appropriate form of evaluation, or to develop the research protocol with the service providers who may be too busy trying to survive to consider whether or not their survival actually allows a worthwhile service to be continued. The implementation of the NHS and Community Care Act 1990 will have appeared like this to many people. It may be wise to allow the dust to settle in some parts of the service, although others may wish to harness the objective judgement of skilled evaluators to their cause, and thus strengthen their probability of survival. Thus times of radical change can also provide opportunities for health technology assessment, but the opportunities will be most fruitful for the politically adept.

Statistical considerations

Two statistical issues are of particular importance in the context of technology assessment. These are *meta-analysis* and *observer bias*. These will be considered briefly below and picked up again in a more general context in Chapter 11.

Meta-analysis

Every professional faced with deciding about appropriateness needs to know how to find and recognize competent trials, and to combine the information from them to form an overall judgement. Only good-quality trials can be combined. Timeliness may be one criterion of quality. Timely technology assessment articles usually appear in journals first, but are they of any use? Their quality can be assessed at two levels:

1. At a relatively simple level, the vocabulary used can be checked: do the terms sensitivity, specificity, false positive, false negative, accuracy, predictive value occur? A relatively unskilled reader could rapidly sort out articles (and often they are all too few) which contained these terms.
2. At a higher level, readers can then question whether the statistical analyses of the distribution of quantitative readings were appropriate, whether the participants were 'blinded', whether observer error was measured, and whether the technology under assessment was randomized (see pp. 95–107). Although this part of the assessment will take considerably more skill, there may actually be precious little to discover, as suggested in a recent article by Cooper and colleagues.[17]

Thereafter, more detailed evaluation of the literature can be carried out, and further advice should be taken, particularly with respect to the statistical techniques required for meta-analysis.

Observer bias

Observer bias is of particular relevance to technology assessment. A useful approach is described by John Grant,[18] and although it is not appropriate for us to describe it here in detail, it is useful to emphasize his underlying idea: the concept of *proportion of agreement*. Measuring the proportion of agreement between observers can clarify why a technology is not having the impact expected of it. If observers vary widely in their interpretation of machine readings or electrical tracings, then it would not be surprising if clinical evaluations eventually proved disappointing. New technologies may be particularly vulnerable to poor inter-observer agreement; a measure of this is obviously an essential part of any health care technology evaluation.

Conclusion

In conclusion, the assessment of technology in health care demands all the skills already described for evaluation generally and some special insights. The process shares techniques used for quality assessment generally, but with some different emphases (see, e.g. Klazinga).[19] A yearning for miracles to change the outcome of some of our most sick and vulnerable should not preclude an intelligent appraisal of whether the technology really can achieve more good than harm (see, e.g. Elliot).[20] All senior NHS staff have a responsibility not to delay the benefits of health technologies, but they must also ensure that money and lives are not wasted by an unqualified enthusiasm for the novel and a disregard for control and consideration.

Chapter 11

Important methodological issues

Introduction

This chapter explores issues connected with the design and analysis of studies. The topics mentioned elsewhere in the book are developed and some new ideas introduced. We have brought together matters which are rarely juxtaposed in standard texts. We suggest that research methodology *per se* has an intrinsic unity and is part of the discipline of medical information science, which in turn should be regarded as applied epistemology (the theory of knowledge) rather than a collection of contributions from diverse disciplines such as statistics, clinical science, the social sciences, etc.

Measurement

The primacy of theory

In everyday life, responses to the world around us are dictated by beliefs about what that world is and how its parts interact with each other and with us. The results of our actions may accord with expectations, in which case those results were predictable from prior beliefs. When results and expectations diverge, we are forced to reappraise our beliefs about the world.

So it is in science. When investigators engage in any study, they must start with some prior beliefs about the system under examination. Those beliefs may be quite tenuous, i.e. they give only general or qualitative predictions about how the system responds in certain circumstances. On the other hand, they may be sufficiently clearly articulated to form a theory capable of very specific predictions. The point is that only when there are beliefs (or theory) to direct our thoughts, are we able to identify important elements of the system under examination. Then we can concentrate effort on understanding how they interrelate. Furthermore, this direction of thought determines what may be presumed observable in the system and how an observation might be recorded, i.e. what is measurable and what, if any, properties of numbers (see Scales of measurement, pp. 150–1) may be attached to the measurement. *Measurement is the means by which attributes of the 'real' world are linked with conceptual models (theories).*

Without the conceptual model, investigators would not know what to measure; if haphazardly they did take measurements (or, strictly, go through procedures which have the formal appearance of being measurements), the results of those measurements would have no meaning. Consider a hospital ward: simple observation reveals that patients come in, stay for varying times and leave; there is usually a fixed number of beds. Suppose we wish to measure the efficiency of the service provided on a particular ward. We could, in the hope that insight would arise, blindly 'measure' everything to hand – the number of doctors, number of nurses, number of patients, number of bed pans, number of light fittings, etc. – but this morass of 'measurements' would reveal little unless we attempted to formulate a conceptual model of the dynamics of a hospital ward. With one such model it becomes apparent that the pertinent measurements are of average bed occupancy, length of stay and turnover interval; indeed, the model specifies how these relate to one another. From the point of view of this model, the number of light fittings is an irrelevance (although this may be highly pertinent to some other model covering other aspects of efficiency).

The foregoing example also illustrates the point that what is a measurement with meaning (or utility) dictated by one theory may within the context of a different theory be an empty procedure. Also, data (i.e. the results of measurements) do not exist in a vacuum – they are *theory-dependent*. That is, potential data do not lie around waiting to be stumbled upon – through our theories we *create* them.

Measuring instruments

An instrument of measurement is the device used to capture data which a theory (conceptual model) specifies as relevant. Examples of instruments include:

- rulers;
- weighing scales;
- sphygmomanometers;
- patient satisfaction questionnaires;
- records clerks coding diagnostic information according to the International Classification of Disease; and
- pairs of radiologists independently assessing mammograms and pooling their findings according to an agreed protocol.

An instrument may have a theoretical basis to its use which is partially independent of the theoretical framework which dictates the utility of the measurement. The use of a sphygmomanometer (to measure blood pressure) is predicated upon the properties of the elastic arterial wall which may be compressed by external pressure; the properties of a column of mercury; the properties of a bag of air; and the likely behaviour of people recording numbers from a scale who may prefer to document figures ending with '5' or '0' rather than a 'precise' reading, etc. These secondary theories and the properties of the real world which they are assumed to mirror determine the degree to which a measuring instrument can actually measure that which it purports to measure; thus in the example just given, there are clear reasons why the direct method of measurement of blood pressure (cannula is an artery connected to a column of fluid) is likely to yield more accurate results than the indirect method (sphygmomanometer).

Operational definition of measurement

A measuring instrument must be operationally defined, i.e. there must be a clear definition of the construction of the instrument and step-by-step instructions for its use. This is necessary to maintain objectivity. In appropriate circumstances, an instrument should yield the same results, within a margin of experimental error, regardless of which suitably trained person uses it.

In general, it is not possible to separate an instrument from the person using it. Both are part of the measurement process. Indeed, as is illustrated by the final example above, an instrument may sometimes consist solely of people forming judgements. In these circumstances, the operational definition is concerned with how that judgement is reached.

Validation of measuring instruments

Validation is the means whereby it is established that an instrument is measuring something adequately close (conceptually and practically) to that which it purports to measure. Validation is generally very difficult. Ultimately, it involves an act of faith. There are some criteria helpful in the assessment of validity.

Construct validity

This is the consistency of the measurement with the theoretical concepts (constructs) concerning the system under study. For instance, if theory dictates that a measurable attribute of a system should change with the passage of time, then actual measurements should change with time. Also, an instrument purporting to measure blood pressure which gave negative readings would be suspect; however, it might merely be biased (see pp. 148–9).

Content validity

This is the degree to which the measurement covers the scope of the system (phenomenon) being studied. For example, a measure of general patient satisfaction should include factors representing satisfaction with care received, accessibility of information, kindness and efficiency of staff, quality of hospital hotel services, etc.

Criterion validity

This is the extent with which the instrument produces measurements consistent with those of another, independent instrument, which purports to measure the same thing or something known to be closely related. Two forms of criterion validity are distinguished:

1. *Concurrent validity*: the criterion and the measurement refer to the same point in time, e.g. when a clinical history of myocardial infarction is found to be consistent with immediate electrocardiogram changes. A special case of seeking concurrent validity is when a new measuring instrument is *calibrated* against another instrument of identical purpose, and perhaps of different design, and which is believed to be valid.

2. *Predictive validity*: the measurement predicts the criterion, e.g. cardiac enzyme levels rise a few days after the initial electrocardiographic events. Predictive validity is a powerful indicator of overall validity, for when a measurement is capable of predicting how some aspect of the system under study will change, it has a clear utility. Sustained raised blood pressure levels are a predictor of the subsequent risk of developing myocardial infarction and stroke; thus regardless of compelling theoretical reasons why blood pressure is an important variable in cardiovascular dynamics, there also are strong pragmatic grounds for measuring blood pressure.

The issue of validation is not merely of relevance to scientists and those studying epistemology – it applies to anyone using an instrument. It is not unusual for someone engaged in evaluative research to use an already validated instrument in somewhat different circumstances to those of its original validation. But it should not be assumed that, for example, an 'off the shelf' patient satisfaction questionnaire will measure precisely what is intended in the circumstances of its proposed use. A newly devised questionnaire must be validated and this requires a special study designed for the purpose.

Minimizing error and bias

An instrument is said to be *biased* if measurements made with it tend to differ in a systematic manner from the 'true' values which a perfect instrument would give. The degree to which repeated measurements differ when an identical result is expected each time represents another form of error. Consider this analogy:

> Suppose there is a marksman who always manages to place a tight cluster of bullet holes on the target board. If this cluster centres on the bull's eye the marksmanship is consistent, accurate and unbiased. If the shots always cluster to the right and below the bull's eye there is a systematic bias which might be remedied by adjustment of the gun-sight. A highly spread cluster of bullets indicates greater inconsistency (*error*) and poorer marksmanship than a tight cluster. However, a less consistent marksman may be unbiased and therefore hit the bull's eye more frequently than the consistent but biased colleague.

In marksmanship, a large bias but tight cluster is likely to score far fewer points than no bias and less accuracy, but in measurement *systematic bias* need not always be cause for concern. If the size of the bias is known, it can be corrected, e.g. subtract a constant value from all readings. If comparisons are being made and *if the same instrument is used for all measurements*, then the bias will disappear because it is the differences in measurements which are important rather than the absolute values.

Bias and error (lack of repeatability) intrinsic to the measuring instrument have to be investigated during validation. Their minimization may require redesign of the instrument. Bias and error may also arise as a consequence of the manner and context of use of the instrument (observer bias). In these circumstances, they may be minimized by proper training and constant checking of persons using it; indeed, it is not safe to assume that people will use even the simplest of instruments (e.g. weighing scales) in a consistent manner.

Problems increase as the element of subjectivity in the use of an instrument increases. The most extreme case is where *people are the instrument*, as for example in the classification of radiographic signs of pneumoconiosis; in this instance, observers have to be extensively trained and must be shown to reach agreement on the majority of cases. All cases, or samples of cases, should be assessed independently by more than one observer. There must be predetermined rules for dealing with disagreements.

Non-medical managers may be surprised at this – that health service staff *do* record weights and blood pressures in a very inconsistent and variable manner when they have all received the same training and respect the need for a disciplined approach. Similarly, the results of many routine investigations are given by specialists *interpreting* what they see; chest X-rays, cervical smears and types of tumour pathology may be unequivocally normal or abnormal, but the majority will be a mix of the normal and the abnormal, and as such the observer's tendency to identify normality and abnormality is a well-recognized source of systematic bias. Such bias can be controlled only if the observers are all trained in a similar fashion, and the study design allows comparisons of each observer, in order to quantify any bias that may have occurred.

Recording schedules are less obviously subjective. Nevertheless, they pose difficulties when anything other than simple factual information (e.g. gender, address, civil status) is sought. The demeanour of the questioner and the manner in which the question is put will sometimes influence the nature of the response. Careful staff training and standardization of all procedures are essential.

In some circumstances, simple error – or lack of repeatability – may be minimized by taking repeated measurements. Statistical theory predicts that the averages of repeated measurements are less variable than the individual measurements. In general, the variance (an index of variability or, in this context, of error) of the arithmetic mean (average) measurement equals the variance of individual measurements divided by the number of measurements. This accords with the intuitive idea that the greater the number of repeated measurements, the greater the accuracy of the overall average. Repeated measurement will *not* reduce systematic bias.

Scales of measurement

The outcome of measurement is the recording of some finding or response. This record may take one of several forms: it may be a prose description of what was observed, classification of an entity as being of a particular type, or some numbers. The form in which a measurement may legitimately be recorded is determined wholly by the *theoretical* properties of that being measured. Thus, for example:

- length of hospital stay is recorded in units of whole days;
- waiting lists are integer numbers of people;
- blood pressure is measured in millimetres of mercury (or any equivalent scale of force per unit area), and in theory but not in practice could be recorded to fractions of a millimetre;
- preferences among a range of alternatives in a survey of opinions can be stated as a rank ordering (i.e. first, second, third, etc.) of the alternatives and these ranks may be represented by whole numbers (1, 2, 3, etc.), but it would usually be nonsense to state that the first preference was preferred four times as much as the fourth preference.

Measurement resulting in prose descriptions will not be discussed here. All other measurement results in a recording which uses some of the properties of numbers. Which of these properties is used determines the legitimate methods of statistical analysis and presentation of the data. Thus, for example, an analysis of data on preferences which treats the recordings as if they had the same numerical properties as blood pressure or weight might lead to grave error of interpretation.

There are four kinds, or scales, of numerical measurement:

1. *Nominal scale*: persons or objects are classified, i.e. assigned on the basis of one or more attributes to one of several mutually exclusive and collectively all-inclusive groups. For example, hospital wards may be classified as medical, general surgical, orthopaedic, etc. The groups can be assigned names (e.g. orthopaedic) or numbered as group 1, group 2, etc. When numbers are assigned, no other numerical relationship (e.g. multiplication) between them should be assumed. Incidentally, the process of classification in formal logic and the branch of mathematics known as set theory are a starting point for the development of the theory of numbers, hence our justification for calling classification a numerical property. (Some writers distinguish between dichotomous scales, i.e. only two possible values, and nominal scales - see Abramson.)[1]

2. *Ordinal or ranking scale*: on the basis of some attribute, persons or objects are placed in rank order, i.e. first, second, third, etc. The only numerical relationships permitted between these numbers are those related to classification (i.e. grouping ranks) and ordering, that is greater than (better than), less than (worse than) and equal to; there is no information as to *how much greater* than, etc.

3. *Interval scale*: the numbers assigned represent changes in degree (e.g.

hotter or colder) like a ranking scale, but also quantify the difference in degree. They can be added together, or subtracted from each other; they can be divided into constituent intervals; they may legitimately take fractional values (e.g. have decimal points). Examples of measurements on this scale include temperature in degrees Fahrenheit or Centigrade and scores from psychometric tests (although it can be argued that most psychometric test scores should strictly be on a ranking scale). On this scale, it may properly be said that 60°C is 30°C hotter than 30°C, but it makes no sense to say it is twice as hot. Measurements on the interval scale have an arbitrary zero point; Fahrenheit and Centigrade are equivalent and easily converted one to the other, yet zero degrees Centigrade corresponds to 32 degrees Fahrenheit.

4. *Ratio scale*: this has all the properties of the preceding scales and in addition an absolute zero point. Examples of measurements on this scale are height, weight and blood sugar concentration. It is acceptable to state that one person is twice as heavy as another.

In general, the so-called non-parametric[2] statistical techniques are appropriate for analysing measurements on the nominal and ordinal scales; statistical models describing the properties of measurements on these scales have no characteristic parameters such as the mean or standard deviation. These methods make few assumptions about the structure and numerical properties of the data.

Parametric methods (typically using arithmetic means and variances calculated from the data) are often applicable to measurements on the interval and ratio scales. However, parametric methods usually make assumptions about the nature and distribution of variation in the data. The most common assumption is that the distribution is Normal (Gaussian), i.e. the frequencies of occurrence of narrowly spaced groupings of the measurement are for large samples approximated by a bell-shaped curve. This is illustrated in Fig. 11.1. In this representation, the frequency of occurrence of values of the measurement between, say, 'A' and 'B' portrayed in the figure is proportional to the area under the curve between 'A' and 'B'.

If assumptions about the distribution cannot be justified, then 'distribution free' methods must be resorted to. These frequently entail analysing the data as if they had only the properties of a lower scale (e.g. ranking) and in the process some information inherent to the data is sacrificed.

As an aside, we note that just as what is measurable is determined by *theory* (see pp. 145–6), so also is the scale of measurement. Consider eye colour: if colour is equated to the frequency of light waves rebounding from the iris, then it can be measured on any of the scales listed above because frequency is on a ratio scale. However, if the measurement of eye colour is prompted by a study of Mendelian genetics, then a nominal scale is theoretically the *only* appropriate scale of measurement. This is because Mendelian genetics is intrinsically particulate, it deals with the effects of combinations of individual genes each of which is supposed to exert a specific *discrete* influence on the characteristics observed; these lead us to suppose that the expressed outcome is measurable in

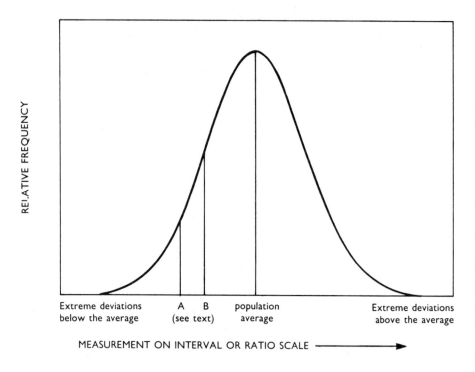

Fig. 11.1 The bell-shaped curve of the Normal distribution.

terms of groups of contiguous frequencies of light, i.e. colours such as blue and brown. However, if the long discredited blending theory of inheritance were being tested, it might make sense to measure eye colour on a ratio scale.

Composite measurements

Investigators frequently try to simplify the task of interpretation by combining a set of measurements into one composite score. This final score should be regarded as the end-point of a single measurement process; that is, the sub-measurements and the manner of their combination forms a single measuring instrument.

There is an infinity of ways by which a set of numbers derived from sub-measurements in the scoring instrument may be combined to give the final score, for each component may be weighted by a different positive or negative number. The choice of these weights is crucial. Thus, if composite scores are to be used, then not only should the component sub-measurements be validated and their scales determined, but also the end score should be validated and its scale determined. For example, if a dependency score is being constructed, it is necessary to demonstrate its utility, i.e. whether it adequately specifies the present need for services or predicts future need.

As an example of some of the complexities that can arise, consider the simplest case: the combination of 'yes/no' responses. Ways of scoring the individual responses include those displayed in Table 11.1. Clearly, methods (a) and (b) are equivalent to each other and so are (c) and (d). However, methods (a), (c) and (e) make entirely different assumptions about the relative values of 'yes' and 'no' responses. The consequences of these differences become apparent when scores from a series of yes/no responses are combined by addition. Under method (a), 'no' responses contribute nothing to the overall total. Under method (c), each 'no' response cancels a 'yes' response. Under method (e), two 'no' responses are required to cancel a 'yes' response. This is illustrated with the fictitious data in Table 11.2, which show the responses from one individual to five questions.

Table 11.1   Examples of scoring systems (see text)

(a)	Yes =	1	No =	0
(b)	Yes =	0	No =	1
(c)	Yes =	1	No =	-1
(d)	Yes =	-1	No =	1
(e)	Yes =	2	No =	-1

If further assumptions had been made about the relative weights given to the scores for individual questions, the picture would become even more confusing.

Table 11.2   Scores by different methods (see also Table 11.1)

Original data		Method				
		(a)	*(b)*	*(c)*	*(d)*	*(e)*
Q1	Yes	1	0	1	-1	2
Q2	No	0	1	-1	1	-1
Q3	Yes	1	0	1	-1	2
Q4	No	0	1	-1	1	-1
Q5	No	0	1	-1	1	-1
Overall score		2	3	-1	1	1

There is a number of statistical tools (e.g. discriminant analysis, principal component analysis and factor analysis) which help in the construction of composite measures. These are complicated and easily abused; discussion of them is beyond the scope of this book. However, a word of warning: there is a plethora of scoring systems (for dependency, general health, psychometric measures, health care needs, social disadvantage, etc.) being hawked around and some have become fashionable – do not assume they have been properly validated. Further discussion of composite measures may be found in Abramson.[1]

At this point, a final warning is opportune on the dangers of making unfounded assumptions about the scale of a measured quantity. This will be illustrated through a fictitious example. Let it be supposed that a psychologist has developed a new instrument for measuring individuals' innate tendency towards aggression. Let it further be supposed that like many other psychometric instruments the resulting scores *appear* to be on an interval scale. Now suppose that there is a deity that can penetrate the inner workings of the mind. This deity can measure aggressive tendency on a ratio scale. Figure 11.2 shows the values of aggression known to the deity and the corresponding values measured by the instrument. (For simplicity, it is assumed that measurements by the instrument are wholly reproducible, etc.) It is clear that at the lower end of the scale, there is a simple linear relationship between the score and the 'true' value (AB and ab on the respective axes of the graph). However, whereas the score changes little between the values B and C, the true value changes considerable (interval bc). The position is reversed with respect to changes between C and D, and the corresponding interval cd on the other axis. Clearly, even if the true value is on a ratio scale, the score cannot be. Moreover, whether the true value is on a ratio or interval scale, the score cannot be on either; for the ratio of intervals along the vertical axis (e.g. ratio of BC to CD) is not the same as the ratio of corresponding intervals on the horizontal axis (e.g. bc to cd). Thus, it would be prudent for our fictitious psychologist to treat the measurement scale as, at best, ordinal, until such time as detailed validation justifies otherwise.

As suggested in Chapter 5, it is often useful to talk through the implications of the numerical values which may have been assigned to various answers; this can aid an understanding of the issues involved. Also, as stated in Chapter 3, do take statistical advice at an early stage in developing the evaluation protocol.

Data coding and storage

Data are recorded after each measurement is made. Thus, for example, with an interviewer-administered recording schedule, the interviewer will record each response as it is elicited. Data can be recorded on paper, orally on a tape-recorder or be typed into a portable computer. The general principles of data handling are the same for each. The discussion will concentrate on data recorded initially on paper. It will be assumed that, subsequently, the data will be transferred into a computer.

The task of handling data is simplified if well-designed forms are used and if attention is given at an early stage of the study design to how the data will be made intelligible to a computer. Computers recognize alphabetical characters and numbers but in general numerical coding is the easiest to handle during analysis. Sometimes data can be recorded directly in a form suitable for

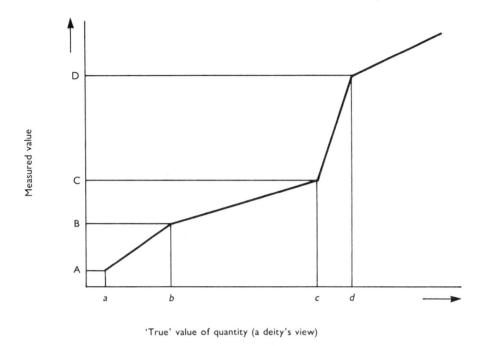

Fig. 11.2   Measurement scales may not be what they appear (see text).

transference to a computer. Usually it is necessary, particularly with questionnaires, to have an intermediate stage of coding. Thus, with a questionnaire, the respondent or interviewer will fill in answers or tick options from a list. Subsequently, someone will have to interpret the responses and transfer them into a format acceptable to the computer. The resulting codes are usually written down for someone else to enter into the computer later. It is convenient if the computer codes can be placed on the original questionnaire, perhaps in a margin reserved for 'office use only' and containing coding boxes ready to receive the codes. The set of coding boxes for one datum is known as a field. The set of fields on the form constitute a record.

The allocation of codes to data is generally straightforward. Examples are given below:

1. *Subject identifiers*. To protect confidentiality, the names and addresses of human subjects are not entered into computer databases unless there are compelling reasons to do so. Generally, each subject is allocated a unique study number. If it should prove necessary to marry together several forms (records) for the same subject or to update the computer record at a later date, it is

prudent to use more than one identifier because a simple typing error in a sole identifier could invalidate the entire record. Additional unique identifiers might include hospital number or NHS (UK) number, but in theory, if not in practice, these lessen confidentiality. Supplementary identifiers which are not unique can be helpful, e.g. postcode (or ZIP) and data of birth.

2. *Polychotomous data.* Gender, 'yes/no' responses and choices from a fixed list of alternatives are examples of polychotomous data. The various alternatives can be coded 1, 2, 3, etc.

3. *Data on interval and ratio scales.* If these never contain a decimal point there is no problem, record them as they are. Numbers with decimal points have to be handled carefully. The decimal point can be recorded explicitly or made implicit by the position of the numbers. The latter arises when, say, four coding boxes are allocated to a number which may contain up to four digits, one of which occurs after a decimal point. In this example, the decimal point is not necessarily displayed on the coding form but is implied between the third and fourth boxes. People coding data have to be careful to ensure that whole number parts always go in the first three boxes even when there is nothing beyond the decimal point. It is good practice to code, say, 27 as 0270 rather than as 27 preceded and followed by an empty box.

4. *Age.* Age should not be recorded. What is required is date of birth. The ages of all subjects, at a specified date, can be calculated on the computer. The specified date may be a notional study date or the recorded date on which the information was elicited.

5. *Dates.* Dates should be allocated six coding boxes, or four if the year is implicit. The format in the UK is 2 boxes for day, 2 boxes for month (1–12) and two boxes for year (i.e. 1992 recorded as 92). In the USA and some other parts of the world, dates are recorded in a different order, i.e. as month, then day and year. Beware of computer packages which make assumptions foreign to your custom.

6. *Not known.* Sometimes during the administration of questionnaires, respondents are unable to answer a question. Coding schemes should allow for this possibility. This is not the same as missing data (see below) because a response has been attempted although it may not be very helpful.

7. *Missing data.* Missing data arise when a particular measurement has not been attempted or is impossible. It is not good practice to leave the fields for missing data blank: slips can occur during data entry to a computer which lead to data being assigned to the wrong place. Missing data in each data field should be allocated a specific code indicating 'not available' or 'unobtainable'. This is quite different from 'I forgot to fill in the boxes'. The computer can be told about this code later. Figure 11.3 illustrates coding schemes for each of these circumstances.

Entering data onto a computer is no longer restricted by the requirement to punch everything onto paper tape or eighty column cards. Hence records (a set of fields) can be of any length. A clerk can enter data directly from coding sheets to a terminal. Some statistical packages and database programs assist the user

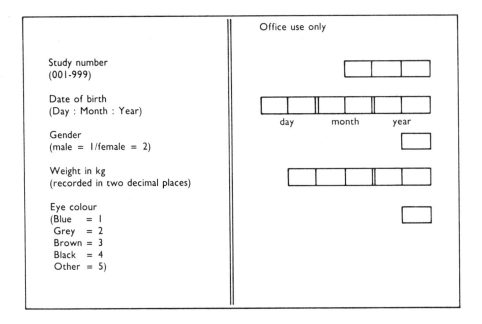

Fig. 11.3 Illustration of coding boxes.

to set up elegant data entry screens. Appropriate programming also allows simple checks to be made of the data as they are entered and errors to be flagged. For instance, if all subjects are known to be aged more than 64 years, an inappropriate birth date will be refused acceptance by the computer. More sophisticated checking can look for consistency among related data items, e.g. females should not be recorded as having had a prostatectomy.

Variation

Measurement error, i.e. variation intrinsic to the measuring instrument, has been discussed and it is evident that steps can be taken to control it. However, even with perfect instruments, considerable variation is to be expected between measurements on a collection of study units even when they are all exposed to the same influences. This is particularly so when research is conducted on biological material (including humans and their institutions). An understanding of sources of variation, of how they can be minimized and of how inferences may be drawn in their presence is the major contribution of statistical theory to the design and analysis of studies. In this section, the nature of variation and the control of variation will be explored. How inferences may be drawn is discussed in the sections on statistical significance and confidence intervals.

Levels of variation

Variation is more easily understood and controlled when it is recognized that it occurs at various levels in a study and that the variation at each higher level is a combination of variations from lower levels. This is best explained by a concrete example: consider a (fictitious) study of the differences in blood pressure between two populations (e.g. women in Scotland and women in Japan).

First, we need to be clear how any difference, if it exists, is to be quantified. If large samples were obtained of Scottish and Japanese women and the blood pressure from every individual measured, then substantial variation would be found between the blood pressures of the women within each sample. This variation would be such that many women would have blood pressures near to their sample average and progressively fewer would have blood pressure that departed further and further above or below the average, i.e. a near bell-shaped (Gaussian) distribution. Moreover, some Scots would have blood pressures greater than most Japanese and vice versa. These distributions are illustrated in Fig. 11.4.

Clearly, if a difference is expected between the populations, it will not be of a simple kind such as 'all Scottish blood pressures are higher than all Japanese pressures'. That is obvious from Fig. 11.4. What it will be sought to infer is that

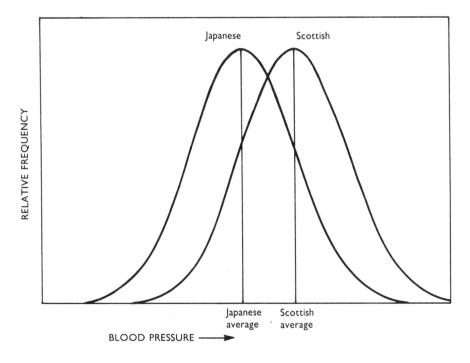

Fig. 11.4 Blood pressure distributions in two populations of women.

the average blood pressure of the Scots differs from the average blood pressure of the Japanese. A crucial decision will be whether any observed difference between the sample averages represents a true difference in the average blood pressures in the populations from which the samples were drawn. This decision will be influenced by the amount of variation (or error) present in the sample averages. This general principle applies to all studies of group differences.

Leaving aside the issue of measurement error, the question arises as to why the blood pressures in either sample vary at all. This is biological variation: it is a statistical manifestation of the fact that people differ. But why do they differ? It has to be presumed that there are underlying factors which determine blood pressure and that some of these are intrinsic to individuals (e.g. genetic) and others a consequence of the circumstance in which they live (e.g. lifestyle habits). If some of these factors were known, it would be possible to draw samples of people who are homogeneous with respect to them. It would be found that the distributions of the blood pressures of these people around their common averages would be less disperse (i.e. show less variation) than the distribution for the entire population around its average. In other words, biological variation is a measure of ignorance of the myriad factors which have influence on the attribute under study; the best research can hope to do is identify major factors which account for a substantial proportion of the general variation.

Not only do blood pressure measurements differ between people, but they also differ *within* the same individual from day to day, hour to hour and minute to minute. So what is meant by an individual's blood pressure? Ideally, there should be a profile of an individual's blood presure over a typical few days; this would give information about the general level of their blood pressure (average) and of how much it varies around that level. In practice, one or more 'samples' of their blood pressure are taken and the profile average inferred from them.

Suppose that a *single* reading of blood pressure is taken on each of the Scots and Japanese in the samples. The final averages of the samples will contain uncertainties contributed by all of the following:

1. Measurement error, i.e. due to inaccurately calibrated sphygmomanometers, using inappropriate cuff sizes, inadequately trained observers, etc.
2. Within-person variation, i.e. the pressure at the time at which the reading was taken was not exactly the long-term average for the subject.
3. Between-person (biological) variation. Also, biological variation may differ between the two populations. This latter would be illustrated by the bell-shaped curves in Fig. 11.4 being of different widths.
4. Sampling variation: a different pair of samples would have contained different people who may have shared fewer, or more, general characteristics with the populations from which the samples were drawn.

The first, second and fourth components of the final variation in the sample averages are amenable to control by the investigator. Measurement error will be reduced by taking the average reading of repeated measurements on the same occasion. Within-person variation may be reduced by repeating measurements on separate days. Sampling variation may be reduced by drawing larger samples.

Because variation is additive and always positive, extra precision at a higher level cannot undo variation or errors introduced at a lower level. *Thus, contrary to what is sometimes supposed, taking larger samples than one otherwise might do does little to ameliorate the effects of errors in a defective measurement procedure.* It is almost certainly not cost-effective. The extent to which it is sought to control the various levels of variation should depend upon their potential contributions to the overall variation.

In Chapter 7, it was pointed out that in some studies it is possible to eliminate between-person variation. This occurs when a subject acts as their own control (or comparison), e.g. left and right hands treated differently for a skin complaint. Strictly, this procedure does not eliminate all between-person variation because there remains the variation between persons in their responses to the treatment (technically this is the person/treatment interaction). The reader is referred to statistical texts for further discussion of these matters.

Regression towards the mean

Regression towards the mean is a well-documented phenomenon which manifests itself in many ways. For instance, the children of intelligent parents tend *on average* to be dimmer than their parents and the children of the dim tend to be brighter than their parents. Similar findings occur for other genetically influenced biometric characteristics, e.g. height. Regression towards the mean can also arise in other contexts and, if unrecognized, lead to serious mis-interpretation of study findings.

The phenomenon will be observed when a characteristic which varies from time to time in individuals is measured repeatedly in those individuals who at first examination lay towards one end of the usual range of variation, i.e. the re-examination of those who are 'extreme'.

Suppose a large population is screened for raised blood pressure and all those with high pressures (e.g. above 100 mmHg diastolic) selected for follow-up. On a subsequent re-examination of that group, their average blood pressure will almost certainly have fallen. The reason for this is that some of the people in the group would have individual averages (as measured over a period of time) which fall below 100 mmHg but on the day of their initial examination their blood pressures were in the higher part of their individual ranges of variation and happened to fall above 100 mmHg; on re-examination, it may be expected that the blood pressures of these people will lie elsewhere in their individual ranges and are likely to be less extreme, and thus the group average will fall.

If investigators had tried a new therapy on this selected high blood pressure group and did not have a comparison group treated differently, then the phenomenon of regression towards the mean would have led them to overestimate the benefits of their therapy. The considerations of this section apply to measurements of all attributes in which *within-person* variation is manifest.

Spurious correlation

There is a phenomenon of *spurious correlation* which is of similar origin as regression towards the mean. This has occurred when investigators have sought to show a relationship between the initial value of some measurement (often blood pressure) on an individual and the change in value on repeated measurement, i.e. final minus initial value correlated to initial value. To seek to do this is natural: it is an attempt to show that people with the most extreme measurements respond the most to treatment. However, it can be shown that if the initial and final values are taken as *random* numbers, the procedure of relating change to initial value will induce a correlation of about − 0.7, i.e. if change is plotted against initial value the points will cluster quite closely around a line sloping downwards from left to right (see Fig. 11.5).

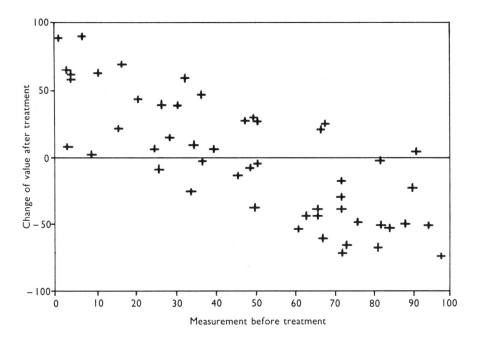

Fig. 11.5 An illustration of spurious correlation. Initial and final measurements consist of random digits between zero and 99.

This phenomenon is fun to verify on a personal computer. It is a logical property of numbers, which has nothing to do with any biological relationship being sought; indeed, it will obscure a biological relationship. The remedy is to relate the arithmetic mean (average) of initial and final readings to the change (difference); this does not induce spurious correlation (see Fig. 11.6). Oldham[3] discusses this further.

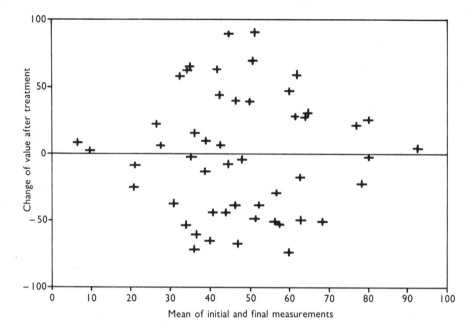

Fig. 11.6   Spurious correlation removed (cf. Fig. 11.5). Initial and final measurements consist of random digits between zero and 99.

Random numbers

Random numbers are employed by persons setting up randomized controlled trials, sampling strategies and simulation studies. In randomized control trials (see pp. 95–107), they assist in gaining an unbiased allocation of patients to treatment groups. In sampling (see pp. 164–9), they assist in drawing a representative sample from a population. In simulation studies, they help to construct models of reality in which the entities under study follow prescribed chances of certain events (simulation is not discussed further in this book).

The concept of randomness is elusive and for the sake of our discussion we shall define a long sequence of digits between 0 and 9 as being near enough random if each of the following conditions holds:

1. Each digit occurs overall on approximately one-tenth of occasions.
2. It is impossible to predict (correlate) one consecutive sub-sequence of the digits from another.
3. It is impossible to predict (correlate) sequences of non-consecutive digits from other such sequences.

Random numbers can be derived from physical processes leading to random outcomes. Various devices have been used. One is to thoroughly mix objects and draw them one at a time as is done with numbered balls at a bingo hall. Another is to rely on the apparently random behaviour of certain electronic circuitry as is done by ERNIE, the British premium bond computer. Both methods demand an act of faith that the underlying process is fundamentally random; this is better justified for ERNIE than for bingo balls but both are adequate for their respective purposes. Coin tossing is not reliable.

It is a remarkable fact that certain repetitive arithmetical operations on numbers, which by definition are inherently fully predictable, can yield sequences of digits which pass a battery of mathematical tests of randomness. These pseudo-random number generators are easily implemented on microcomputers. The user initializes the generator with a haphazardly chosen seed number. Then a sequence of pseudo-random numbers of any desired length can be generated by repeated invocations of the generator. However, a word of caution: some random number generators provided with proprietary software packages have very poor randomness properties or can generate only relatively short sequences before repeating themselves; they sacrifice quality for speed. This will not usually matter for randomized controlled trials or sampling but can invalidate simulation work. If a good generator is essential, it is best to implement one of a number of published and well-tested routines.[4]

Random numbers can be generated and put to use solely within a computer. However, it is sometimes useful to have them in printed lists. Those with computers can print their own but also there are published tables of random numbers. Typically, a page of random numbers would be laid out in rows and columns thus:

59236	67258	48682	18391	07735	12429	83817
73705	82265	07231	42224	71175	87258	31387
37306	81751	14825	18477	64706	39673	51064

When using such tables, a starting page and a starting row and column on the page should haphazardly be selected. Ideally, previously used pages should be ignored.

When preparing to allocate randomly patients to one of two treatments and with a fifty-fifty chance of their being in either, proceed as follows:

1. Take the first digit at the selected starting place, say the beginning of row two in the example above.
2. If the number is 0, 1, 2, 3 or 4, denote it as treatment A. Otherwise denote it as treatment B. In our example, '7' denotes treatment B.
3. Write the allocation, treatment A or B, on a card and put it in a sealed envelope and number the envelope '1'.
4. Go to the *next* consecutive digit, in this case '3' (which denotes treatment A), and repeat the process. Label the second envelope '2'.
5. Continue *systematically* through the table until sufficient allocations have been made. It is permissible to go down columns rather than along rows, but one or other route should be taken consistently.

6. When patients attend the clinic and have consented to enter the trial, open the next unopened envelope from the ordered stack of envelopes. Obviously, it is desirable that the person who prepared the envelopes not be the person allocating the patients.

In other contexts such as sampling, random numbers ranging beyond 0 to 9 are required. Suppose that random numbers between 1 and 300 are sought. Proceed as follows:

1. From the selected starting point, e.g. beginning of second row, take the number formed by the first three digits, e.g. 737. If this is not zero (000) and not greater than 300 accept it, otherwise discard it. In our example, the first triple set of digits is discarded.
2. Proceed to the next consecutive triple and repeat the procedure. In our example, this is 058 (i.e. fifty-eight) and is accepted.
3. Continue systematically along rows (or down columns).

Sampling

When the number of people or things under investigation (the *study population*) is large, it is usually impracticable to examine them all. In circumstances such as these, a sample is taken and from the properties of the sample inferences are made about the population from which the sample was drawn. If these inferences are to be valid, the sample must *represent* the characteristics of the population. Four considerations determine whether a sample is likely to be representative:

1. A clear definition of the population being sampled and a well-stated means (*sampling frame*) for identifying potential sample members.
2. The sampling strategy, i.e. the method by which sample members are selected.
3. The size of the sample. Small samples can reflect only coarse features of the population; subtlety requires large samples.
4. The proportion of those selected to be in a sample who respond to the request for information; this is commonly known as the *response rate* but is more correctly termed the response *ratio*.

Sampling frames

A sampling frame is a list of all the members (e.g. people, things, hospitals) of the population from which the sample is to be drawn. For a particular study, there may be several potential sampling frames and each will carry various advantages and disadvantages with regard to accessibility, coverage, being up to date, ease and cost of use. For samples from the general population, the following are some of the potential sampling frames:

1. *The electoral register*. This omits those not eligible to vote (e.g. children); some people fail to register (e.g. gypsies); it can be inaccurate towards the end of the year, especially for highly mobile population groups (e.g. students). However, the register is a public document; copies may be bought, in computer readable form if desired; and it is available in public reference libraries. Electoral registers cover defined geographical areas.

2. *General practitioner age/sex registers*. These are becoming increasingly useful. However, inaccuracies can be considerable, because not everyone need register with a doctor, and because it may take a long time for people who move or change doctors to be erased from the register. Unfortunately, GP lists do not, indeed cannot, coincide with defined geographical areas. Tabulation by age and gender greatly simplifies the selection of samples from age or gender sub-groups of the general population. Many practice registers are stored on computer and this makes the drawing of samples particularly easy. Increasing numbers of Family Health Service Authorities (FHSAs) are maintaining central computer registers of patients in practices under their supervision. Permission must be sought from GPs before an FHSA will allow access to its registers.

3. *Council community charge registers*. Current legislation does not allow them to be made available to researchers; moreover, these registers will soon become defunct.

4. *Telephone directories*. This can be a hopelessly biased sampling frame for the general population as possession of a telephone correlates with affluence. Even as a sampling frame of telephone users it is out of date, and biased because it omits ex-directory premises. Nevertheless, the telephone directory is widely used, especially in the USA. It should be used as a sampling frame of last resort or in circumstances where the biases are unimportant.

Examples of sampling frames in other contexts include:

1. Professional persons may be sampled from their professional registers, e.g. state registered nurses. Such registers are usually reasonably up-to-date.
2. Out-patient attenders at a particular hospital could be sampled from all those listed as having appointments during, say, a particular week.
3. In-patients could be sampled from a list of all those known to have been in hospital at midnight on particular days. These lists would most accurately be obtained from administrative records. Retrospectively, if other records are not accessible, the sampling frame could be derived from Korner index files via patient hospital numbers.
4. British state-sector hospitals can be identified from the NHS Yearbook.
5. Registered nursing homes can be identified from local authority or NHS records.

Sampling strategies

There are many possible strategies. The following are some – not necessarily mutually exclusive – possibilities:

1. *Simple random sampling*: all members of the sampling frame are allocated unique numbers in sequence starting from one. Suppose the sampling frame contains 7128 subjects. Then a series of four-digit pseudo-random numbers is obtained from published tables or generated on a computer (see pp. 162-4). These numbers are examined in sequence and each that corresponds to a number in the range of the sampling frame means that the subject with that number is included in the sample. The process continues until a sample of requisite size is obtained. If a particular subject's number is selected more than once, the second and subsequent selections are ignored (sampling without replacement). Simple random sampling has the property that all *samples* of the same size are *equally likely to be selected* and the statistical theory for dealing with this kind of sample is straightforward and well developed.

2. *Stratification*: sometimes investigators wish to be sure that reasonable numbers of persons with particular characteristics are represented within the sample. Thus, although simple random samples would *on average* have equal numbers of males and females from a population in which the genders are equally represented, any particular instance is unlikely to be evenly balanced. If even balance is important, the population may be stratified into males and females and separate simple random samples drawn from each stratum. Sometimes it may be desired that the final sample gives one stratum greater weight than it has in the population. A simple random sample of people aged over 70 years would have proportionately few persons aged 85 and above. To get good representation of the latter, it would be feasible to take, say, a 1 in 50 sample of the young elderly and a 1 in 10 sample of the old elderly.

3. *Systematic sampling*: for example, for a 1 in 20 sample take the 5th, 25th, 45th, 65th, etc., persons from the sampling frame. This is a simple method but not generally regarded as safe. Subtle bias may arise if in some way the numbering system in the sampling frame happens to correlate with some characteristics of the population.

4. *Multi-stage sampling*: sometimes there is no natural sampling frame for the population under study and it may not be feasible to create one by going out and identifying all members. Suppose that a national sample of ward cleaners was sought: the first stage might be to draw a sample of hospitals (perhaps stratified by type) from a list of all hospitals; next each of the selected hospitals would be approached and ward cleaners identified from the payroll; finally, within each hospital samples of the cleaners would be selected. This is an example of a two-stage sampling strategy.

5. *Quota sampling*: this entails selecting pre-set numbers of people possessing specified characteristics. For example, a survey assistant might be instructed to go to a shopping centre and administer a questionnaire to 10 persons in each of the following categories: white-collar workers, blue-collar workers, unemployed and students. On approaching likely candidates, identified by appearance, the assistant would ask some initial questions to verify their hunch and only administer the questionnaire if the candidate fulfilled their needs. Quota sampling is commonly used by market researchers and opinion pollsters. There may be a place for it in consumer surveys on health

services but there are many potential biases to mislead the unwary. There is a, perhaps apocryphal, tale of the opinion pollster whose quota sample was almost unanimously in favour of legalizing prostitution; the interviewer had unwittingly been sited just round the corner from a bawdy house.

Response ratio

This is the proportion of subjects from whom information is sought who actually respond (give information). Rarely will the response in a large survey be 100%, but the *best investigators in the most carefully designed studies often achieve between 95 and 99% response.*

The key problem in the interpretation of any survey which does not achieve 100% response is guessing the extent to which *non-respondents* differ in important characteristics from respondents and the degree to which this difference biases the findings. Consider the following fictitious example:

A survey of morbidity among people aged 70 years and over was conducted. The elderly were randomly sampled from general practice age/sex registers and invited to attend special clinics at health centres. Various measurements of morbidity were made and scored such that no morbidity (or deficit) scores 10 and high morbidity scores 0.

Table 11.3 portrays the results which might be obtained for different levels of response.

Table 11.3   Outcome by level of response (fictitious data): Median scores

Response %	Mean age	Vision	Mobility	Mental acuity
10	72.7	9	9	10
30	74.9	7	8	9
50	76.2	6	7	8
70	77.3	5	6	7
80	78.1	4	5	6
100	78.6	3	4	4

In this example, it is obvious that those with the greatest morbidity or disability tend to be those who find it most difficult to respond. This difficulty correlates with age. Hence investigators content with a low response would get a wrong impression of the pattern of morbidity among the elderly.

Response may be maximized by the following methods:

1. Taking care in the manner by which potential study subjects are aproached: clear friendly invitation; intelligible explanation of reasons for study; assurance of confidentiality (where applicable); being seen as competent; causing little inconvenience to subjects.

2. Do not take 'no' for an answer too easily. It is possible to apply gentle persuasion without being boorish or infringing someone's civil liberties.
3. Multiple mail-shots of postal questionnaires. Each invitation letter should differ from the last and stress the value placed on receiving information from the subject. Try to make the correspondence 'personal', i.e. address to the person by name (not the 'occupier') and if feasible have letters individually signed.
4. Enclose a stamped addressed envelope marked 'Urgent and Confidential' with each mailing.
5. Bribery: few would take offence at being given a free pen with which to fill out a questionnaire or some other gift of little intrinsic value.
6. Send a fieldworker round to the homes of those who do not respond.
7. In tight communities where general backing for a study has been obtained, it is possible to 'shame' the recalcitrant few into participation.
8. Send a summary of the final results to the respondents. This will prove that the effort made by the respondents was worthwhile and retain goodwill for future studies. For large population studies, it may be more practicable to publicize a summary of the findings, and actions to flow from them, in the local press.

The late Professor Archie Cochrane undertook large longitudinal epidemiological studies in South Wales coal-mining communities which achieved responses in excess of 98%. Before embarking on studies, he solicited the support of community leaders, trades union officials and employers. He sent invitations to individuals and if these were ignored a fieldworker able to relate well to miners and their families would visit the home. If this failed, Cochrane would make a personal visit in his white Jaguar car, such vehicles being a rarity in mining communities, and offer to drive subjects to the survey clinic.

When response is less than 100% it is, nevertheless, often possible to find out something about the characteristics of the non-respondents and quantify the likely extent of bias. For instance, if the sample is drawn from a general practice age/sex register, the GP's case notes will contain some relevant information about non-respondents. Census-derived statistics give an impression of the social characteristics of geographical populations from whom there may be a poor response in population surveys.

As a rule of thumb, 50% response is almost useless and reputable journals are unlikely to publish findings based on such a response unless other factors provide a compelling reason; 70% response is poor and should be interpreted with extreme caution; 80% response is just about adequate and only if something is known about the non-respondents; 90% response is often adequate, but 95% response and above is the standard to be aimed at. Despite the council of perfection it should be borne in mind that a sample does say *something* definite about the respondents. Thus if a patient satisfaction survey with 60% response identifies problems, these are important findings to be followed up; the difficulty is in extrapolating the findings to the entire population from which the sample was drawn. Problems could be over-estimated because persons with complaints were better motivated to respond, or underestimated because people with complaints were too disillusioned with the health service to believe that complaining serves a purpose.

Obtaining a good response can be expensive, but it is an aspect of study design as important as validation of instruments and selection of appropriate sample size. Statistical techniques applicable to random samples are based on the assumption of 100% response. Therefore, investigators must not look to statistical prowess to undo the effects of poor study design and execution.

Study size and inference

For every study with clearly defined objectives, and yielding measurements possessing one or more of the properties of numbers, it is possible to estimate the minimum study size (number of study units) required to give a reasonable chance of there being conclusive results. To do this, the investigator needs prior knowledge or plausible expectations about the magnitude of the effect being studied and of the source and magnitude of variation (e.g. biological variation) among the units upon which measurements are to be made. This knowledge may be gained from a pilot study or from findings from similar studies conducted by others.

Readers wishing to undertake study size calculations should consult a statistician. Here some essential concepts are introduced, an understanding of which will make a statistical consultation more fruitful. Also, by way of examples, the reader will soon be helped to gain some intuition about the sizes of study required to answer certain kinds of question.

Discussion will start with the concept of statistical significance. This is an important tool of inference and an understanding of it is necessary for the notion of study power, which leads to the estimation of desirable study size.

Statistical significance tests

We have stressed repeatedly that every evaluative study must involve comparison. If the indices for comparison are – as most will be – on a numerical scale, then at the end of the study the investigators will be comparing at least one pair of numbers. To make the issue concrete, let it be supposed that the indices for comparison are the proportions of patients satisfied by two different ways of organizing general surgical out-patient clinics. Moreover, it shall be assumed that the study was well designed, properly conducted and that the response was 100%.

Suppose the results showed that 80% of patients were satisfied with one way of organizing general surgical out-patient clinics (method A) and 90% were satisfied with the other (method B). Can it be concluded that method B is superior to method A? On the face of it yes, but in fact we are not yet in a position to make any judgement.

Suppose that these estimates of satisfaction were based on two samples of 10 patients each. No matter how perfectly these samples of patients had been drawn, few people would be happy to conclude that this study proved method B superior to method A. Just by chance those samples could have contained people unrepresentative of clinic attenders and, in any case, samples of 10 are rather small to distinguish between 80% and 90% satisfaction. The importance of sample size is covered in a later section; here we discuss how to deal with the results from the sample.

If this is not clear, consider the tossing of a 'fair' coin, i.e. one for which the chances of heads or tails occurring are equal. Experiment soon indicates that on 10 consecutive tossings it is unusual to end up with exactly five heads and five tails. Six heads and four tails would be unlikely to arouse suspicion that the coin is not fair. On the other hand, nine heads and one tail might, if one were gambling, cause one to harbour suspicions about the owner of the coin. Thus, in the out-patient example, if in reality 80% of *all* patients (not just the samples) were satisfied in *both* clinics, it would not be surprising if two samples of 10 respectively yielded eight and nine responses of satisfaction.

The nub of the issue of statistical interpretation is whether or not observed differences between samples truly reflect underlying differences between the populations from which the samples were drawn. Manifestations of a real difference, if it exists, have to be distinguished from 'fog' or random variation (error) introduced by the sampling and measuring procedures, i.e. the observed difference between the samples is a *combination* of any real difference and random error.

Probability theory describes how random variation behaves. If within the context of a study the nature and distribution of this 'error' is known, or can be estimated, then the contribution of random variation to the observed sample differences can be computed. Consequently, it is possible in a test of *statistical significance* to make a statement about how probable it is that the observed sample difference arose from chance effects alone.

The essence of a statistical significance test is as follows. The investigators set up a *null hypothesis* that in reality there is no underlying difference between the populations, i.e. zero difference. On this assumption and with knowledge of the nature of random variation in the context of the study, they ask themselves 'how likely is it that a difference as great *or greater* than that actually observed could have arisen purely by chance?' Suppose this probability works out as one in five, i.e. if the null hypothesis is true and the study were replicated many times, then on one in five occasions they would observe a difference as great or greater than that actually observed on this occasion. In this circumstance, the investigators would conclude that the difference actually observed would not be unusual as a *chance event*; that is, the study has produced no convincing evidence that one method of organizing an out-patient department is better than the other.

Now suppose that the significance test gave a chance of 1 in 1000. An investigator might reason as follows:

From my assumption (the null hypothesis) I have deduced that it is very unlikely that by chance alone I would observe the difference I actually observed. Rare events do occur, but by definition they occur rarely. Therefore, I may either conclude that my null hypothesis is true and I have observed a rare event, or, because rare events occur rarely, I may conclude that what I observed was not in itself rare but the assumption underlying my calculation was false – that is, I should reject my null hypothesis.

Rejection of the null hypothesis forces acceptance of the *alternative hypothesis* that there is a true underlying difference between the populations from which the samples were drawn, i.e. one method of organizing out-patient clinics is more acceptable to patients than the other. The probability (index of rarity) at which an investigator chooses to reject the null hypothesis is known as the *significance level*. A significance test which leads to rejection of the null hypothesis is said to be *significant* at the stated significance level. To avoid unconscious bias, the significance level should be specified before the data are examined.

Thus, significance tests are decision-making tools which give a dichotomous answer – accept or reject the null hypothesis. The answer determines the decision whether or not to act in the belief that a real difference between the populations has been detected. All decisions are subject to error and the consequences of making a wrong decision must be borne in mind.

The errors associated with significance tests are termed type 1 and type 2 errors. Type 1 errors occur when investigators wrongly conclude that the null hypothesis is false. This is analogous to a false positive result in a medical screening test. This error occurs because rare events do sometimes happen. The probability of a type 1 error is, *by definition*, the significance level chosen for the test. If the chosen level is 5% (probability of 5 in 100), then on 5% of occasions when tests are performed at this significance level a difference of sample averages as large or larger than that observed will occur by chance alone and investigators will wrongly accept the alternative hypothesis. If the consequences of a type 1 error are likely to be serious, a stringent probability level (e.g. 0.1%) should be chosen.

Type 2 errors occur when an investigator incorrectly is led to accept the null hypothesis even though there is a genuine difference between the populations under examination. This is analogous to a false negative result from a medical screening test. Intuitively, it should be clear that if the difference between the populations is small and the sample sizes not large, the random 'fog' from sampling will be of greater magnitude than the underlying difference being sought. This will lead an investigator to conclude, under the assumption that the null hypothesis is true, that the observed difference relative to the 'fog' is compatible with being a chance effect.

The *power* of a significance test is defined as one minus the probability of a type 2 error, i.e. the chance that a type 2 error does not occur. This is the probability that a *specified* minimum real difference between the populations under examination would lead to an observed sample difference which would be deemed statistically significant at a *stated* significance level. If the specified real difference and study size are kept constant, the power of the test declines as significance levels become more stringent.

For example, suppose the *real* patient acceptability of methods A and B for organizing out-patient clinics is 90 and 70% respectively, i.e. a difference of 20 percentage points. A significance test at the 5% level of significance (i.e. type 1 error probability of 0.05) is said to have 90% power against the stated difference if on many replications of the study 90% of these replications lead the investigators to conclude that the *observed* sample difference is significant at the 5% level. The type 2 error of these tests is 10% (i.e. 100% − 90%); alternatively, the type 2 error expressed as a probability is 0.1 (i.e. 1.0 − 0.9).

In reality, an investigator does not know whether there is a real population difference of interesting magnitude, and hence the need for a study. The best that can be hoped is to keep the type 1 and type 2 errors at acceptable levels. The levels chosen depend upon the consequences of the errors. The investigator always has direct control of the type 1 error (significance level), but the type 2 error depends upon the magnitude of the real difference being sought, the significance level and the study size.

Finally, a note on a widespread confusion about the meaning of the term null hypothesis. Too often investigators when pressed to state their study objectives say 'My null hypothesis was . . .'. As should be clear from the discussion above, a null hypothesis is merely a technical device used in significance tests. It is an Aunt Sally put up to be knocked down by the test. A null hypothesis need not coincide with a study objective or scientific hypothesis. Often the null hypothesis that, say, there is no difference between two groups, is the exact opposite of the study hypothesis that there *is* a difference between the groups.

The determination of study size

The determination of the size of a study entails the following steps:

1. Estimation of the nature and magnitude of random variation (error) inherent to the study. This may be deduced from a pilot study.

2. Selection of the principal end-point measures of the study on which the study size calculation will be made. That is, decide which are the crucial measurements that will determine the findings upon which subsequent decisions for practical action will be made.

3. Deciding upon the smallest real difference between the groups being compared which would be of *practical* interest. In the context of health services research, this implies determining before the study is conducted the kinds of clinical or managerial decisions which might be made as a result of the study. In the example of out-patient clinics given in the previous section, management is unlikely to be interested in acting upon findings which demonstrate a five percentage point difference in patients' perceptions of the quality of service but a twenty percentage point difference could be very important.

4. Quantify the consequences of wrongly concluding that a real difference of practical importance exists when in fact it does not. These consequences may be financial or ethical, e.g. not establishing that the 'best' treatment is best. This leads to the desired type 1 error (significance level).

5. Quantify the consequences likely to ensue from not detecting a true difference of the stated magnitude. Again these consequences may be financial or ethical. From these considerations, the type 2 error and power of the study are determined.

6. Quantify the cost of the study under various assumptions about study size. These considerations should also be borne in mind when looking at the consequences of type 1 and type 2 errors. The 'perfect' study is rarely practicable or affordable. Compromises will have to be made somewhere (i.e. size of effect sought, type 1 error and power), but it is important to estimate their effects.

The magnitude of the minimum difference to be detected, the significance level and the power can be plugged into one of a number of standard formulae appropriate for the study at hand and the desirable sample sizes will be estimated.

The sample size estimate will have been made on the assumption that there will be 100% response. If 90% response is anticipated, the numbers should be scaled upwards accordingly. Bear in mind, however, the discussion on pp. 167–9.

We return to the out-patient clinic study and present in Table 11.4 figures on study size given various assumptions about power and significance level. The first two columns of the table show assumptions about the real underlying levels of satisfaction among patients at the two clinics; the study size is the total of two equal samples. The rest is self-explanatory.

Table 11.4 Study size required for a given power at a stated significance level in a survey of patient satisfaction

| True satisfaction | | Power % | Study size at significance level of | |
Method A %	Method B %		5%	1%
50	55	90	4160	5950
		95	5170	7100
50	60	90	1040	1480
		95	1280	1760
50	70	90	250	360
		95	300	420
50	80	90	100	150
		95	120	170
50	90	90	50	70
		95	60	80

The figures in Table 11.4 show that the required study size becomes greater as the precision of the study increases: smaller differences to be detected, smaller type 1 errors and greater power have to be paid for. As another example of the importance of study size and power issues, consider the following.

Let it be assumed that a change in antenatal care and obstetric practice has been proposed which it is believed might reduce perinatal mortality by 20%. Consider a health district in which on average there are 34 stillbirths and deaths in the first week of life among 3500 births per year. This gives a perinatal mortality rate of 9.7 per 1000 live and stillbirths. It is hoped to reduce this to 7.7 per 1000, i.e. a reduction in deaths to 27 per year. Suppose a comparison is to be made between the 'improved' service and an unaltered service in a nearby district which has similar perinatal mortality and annual number of births; this is a simple but not necessarily efficient study design. It can be shown that a study to detect a 20% reduction in perinatal mortality leading to a significance test with a significance level of 5% and power of 90% would require observing *45,000* births in each of the two districts. This would take 13 years. If there were a lot of interest in doing this study, it would be wise to look at ways of recruiting the large number required within a short time-scale, e.g. 12 districts randomly allocated to standard care or the change in care.

In the context of clinical trials, it is widely accepted that a 30% improvement by one treatment compared to another is usually the least that it is feasible to detect. With regard to perinatal mortality, it is unreasonable to expect that any single medical or social intervention will have as great an impact as 20% because efforts to reduce perinatal mortality are already near the point of diminishing returns. In general, even for common diseases like coronary heart disease in middle-aged men, mortality statistics are not suitable outcome measures for small-scale studies conducted in single hospitals or on health authority populations.

In the case of the improvements to the obstetric service, it might be sensible to broaden the criteria of outcome. There could be a move from mortality to morbidity. This would increase the number of morbid events and thus lessen the length of the study. Even so, it is likely that such a study would be too ambitious to undertake in a single hospital because the time-scale would still be long. Furthermore, morbidity lacks the precision of definition of mortality. It is many-faceted; there would be problems in capturing all relevant morbid events; the data would be from differing sources and hard to standardize for quality; morbid events differ in severity and in consequence are hard to pool.

Another possibility would be to measure indices which it is generally agreed reflect the quality of pregnancy, e.g. birth weight. This has the advantage of being universally recorded (with variable accuracy) and of appearing in official statistics which allow comparison between places. In a typical UK health district, it may be feasible to design a study capable of demonstrating a *substantial* change in average birth weight over a period of 2–3 years.

Regardless of how a sufficiently large sample is accumulated, the key feature is that it is the *number* of people or events in the sample which dictates the power of the statistical manipulations applied to the results. It is *not* whether or not the sample represents a sufficiently large proportion of the sampling frame. The number of people or events in a sample is crucial to our being able to say whether or not there are statistically significant differences between groups; it is irrelevant whether that sampling fraction represents 10%, 1% or 0.1% of the population as a whole. Simple random sampling, as already discussed, should help in ensuring that the members of a sample are reasonably representative of the population from which they are drawn: the *size* of the sample determines whether comparisons are statistically robust.

Problems with significance tests

Significance tests have serious limitations. Being simple yes/no decision rules, they lack finesse. A non-significant result should not be taken as meaning that there are no differences of interest between the populations from which the samples were drawn. Perhaps the study was too small to be sufficiently powerful or, perhaps, in a large study, there was a type 2 error. Whether or not findings are formally statistically significant, prudent investigators look at the magnitude of the differences actually observed and explore these within the context of the consistency of their entire data set. Moreover, a statistically significant result does not imply that the difference detected was 'real' (perhaps there was a type 1 error) or, if real, of practical importance.

Multiple significance testing within one body of data poses problems. This usually arises when investigators indulge in *fishing expeditions*. They gather data on many variables but with no clear prior hypotheses and hope that something of interest will emerge. This is bad research. However, even respectable studies may occasion large numbers of measurements and it is tempting to look at these in different ways. Unfortunately, it is a simple consequence of the logic of significance tests that if, say, 100 tests at the 5% level of significance are performed, then on average 5 of those tests will be significant even though there is no underlying difference between the groups from which the samples were drawn.

It is tempting to scour a large series of significance tests and latch onto the statistically significant results. If these are picked out of the context of the non-significant findings and presented as important findings of the study, they may seriously mislead the investigators and others. If a desire for multiple testing must be indulged, then the consequent bias should be minimized by using more conservative significance levels. That is, the nominal level for each test may be 5%, but in fact the decision rule for each test uses an actual significance level of, say, 1%. Thus, although each test will be interpreted as if performed at the 5% significance level, only 1% of the tests will, on average, have resulted in type 1 errors. The reader is referred to statistical texts for details.

There is another serious bias affecting the literature which investigators refer to for knowledge about their field of study. Positive results, i.e. those which are statistically significant, tend to be accepted for publication more easily than negative findings. Because of type 1 errors, a proportion of these positive studies (particularly if they are small) are spurious and these are not counterbalanced in the literature by the negative findings of other studies. Reputable journals should publish positive and negative findings on the proviso that both kinds of study have been demonstrated to be intrinsically powerful enough to detect differences of interest.

The moral of the tale is that significance tests should be used only as a guide in the analysis and interpretation of findings; a slavish adherence to significance testing indicates a thoughtless investigator.

Confidence intervals

When presenting findings about quantities measured on an interval scale, ratio scale or as proportions, it is useful not merely to quote significance levels for observed differences but also to display the range of precision of the estimated quantity. Thus rather than saying that the difference in patient acceptability between two methods of organizing out-patient clinics was ten percentage points and that this was statistically significantly different from zero, it is helpful to show that the range of the estimated difference lies between, say, six and fourteen percentage points with 95% confidence.

The calculation of a confidence interval will not be described here. The interpretation of a 95% confidence interval is as follows. If the study were to be replicated many times and for each replication the 95% confidence interval were calculated, then 95% of those intervals would contain the true (population) value of the quantity being estimated from sample(s). Thus, for any particular study, the true value of the quantity being estimated (e.g. the difference in patient levels of satisfaction) either does or does not lie within the calculated interval and there is no way of knowing which holds. However, one hopes that one's particular realization of the infinite number of possible ways the study might have turned out is an instance of the 95% of studies whose confidence intervals would contain the true value. Note that the confidence intervals from the hypothetical replicate studies would in general differ in central value and distance between the upper and lower limits. This is because each study would provide a different *estimate* of the parameter of interest (e.g. the population mean) and of its standard error (i.e. variability).

A 99% confidence interval gives even greater prospect that a realization of a study will give rise to an interval containing the true value. However, greater confidence has to be traded against a wider confidence interval. One hundred per cent confidence is unattainable, or rather it leads to an uninformative confidence interval which contains the entire range of possible values of the quantity being measured.

For a given amount of intrinsic variation in the study units, the larger the study size becomes the narrower is the confidence interval for any pre-determined level of confidence. This ties in with the intuitive notion that the larger a sample becomes the greater is the precision of the estimate of some quantity in the population from which the sample was drawn.

Confidence intervals are closely related to significance tests. Suppose a

95% confidence interval is constructed for the difference between two sample averages. If this interval encompasses zero difference, then a corresponding significance test at the 5% level of significance would not lead to rejection of the null hypothesis, i.e. the observed difference or a bigger one could have arisen with a chance greater than 5 in 100 when there is no real underlying difference between the populations from which the samples were drawn. If, however, zero difference lies outside the range of the confidence interval, the corresponding significance test would have led the investigator to reject the null hypothesis and conclude that the observed difference reflected a real underlying difference, i.e. the probability associated with the test would be 5 in 100 or less.

The convoluted logic underlying confidence intervals may appear like something from Alice in Wonderland. It appeals to an infinity of studies which, apart from one, happen only hypothetically. However, for practical purposes, there is no harm in thinking of confidence intervals as ranges of precision based on what actually happened. Nowadays, many medical journals demand that, when appropriate, confidence intervals be presented rather than just simple estimates of quantities and significance tests. This is a move we welcome.

Analysis and inference

The foregoing discussion of significance testing and confidence intervals barely touches upon the repertoire of techniques of statistical analysis and inference. Which techniques should be used depends upon the study design, the scales of measurement employed, and the nature of the answers being sought. All evaluative studies lead to some kind of comparison which usually can be interpreted with the aid of simple significance tests or confidence intervals. Some studies of sophisticated design may require a comparison of how one quantity varies with another between one or more groups, e.g. survival patterns with time following differing treatments. Studies in which the effects of several variables are being looked at simultaneously (e.g. survival pattern *vs* drugs), rather than piecewise, require the elaboration of a statistical model to disentangle complicated relationships.

Statistical models are expressed mathematically. They generally consist of two parts: an elaboration of structure and a description of random variation or error. The structural element attempts to reflect the following:

1. The relationships between the study units consequent upon the study design. For instance, if a health promotion technique has been tested on individuals from different factories, then the model must take account of the fact that individuals working in the same factory have something in common which is not shared with individuals in different factories.
2. Relationships that prior knowledge specifies must exist between certain measurable quantities.
3. Hypothesized relationships between measurements or study units which the study is seeking to demonstrate or refute.

During analysis, the structural component of a model may go through several variations as the investigators seek the simplest form capable of summarizing (or 'explaining') the mass of data before them. The random component of the model makes plausible assumptions about the properties of the random variation inherent to the data. Rather than explaining the structure of any relationship present among the data, it attempts to describe the 'fog' which obscures that relationship. Inferences are made about apparent relationships in the light of knowledge of the extent of the fog, i.e. significance tests are performed and confidence intervals computed.

One of the most commonly used statistical models is known as multiple linear regression. It has several variants. Many statistical packages used on microcomputers can perform multiple regression. It is easy for anyone to input data and obtain answers. However, multiple regression is a subtle tool and can easily mislead the unwary.

Those who do not possess statistical skills are advised to keep well away from statistical modelling techniques. However, used with care, these techniques are helpful in bringing forth fine detail from study data. They can also help generate subsidiary hypotheses which might be worth exploring in future studies. It should, however, be borne in mind that in evaluative work which is intended to have practical consequences, the main findings of the study should hit one between the eyes after simple analysis and tabular or graphical presentation of results. Findings which emerge only after arcane statistical incantations should be viewed with suspicion.

Sensitivity analysis

Sensitivity analysis is a technique for testing the robustness of conclusions to changes in the assumptions which led to them. For example, a new service plan may be based in part on quantities estimated from routine data sources and, perhaps, on one or more special studies. It will be known that all the quantities upon which the plan is based are subject to a margin of error. Sensitivity analysis of the plan entails making plausible assumptions about the magnitudes of the errors and seeing whether the implications of the plan (e.g. cost, workload, case-severity, etc.) change much as the underlying quantities are allowed to vary within their ranges of error. The ranges of error of quantities estimated from well-designed studies might be taken from their 95% confidence intervals. For other quantities, the likely ranges of error will be guessed. Sensitivity analysis, sometimes of heroic proportions, is much used by economists.

Meta-analysis

Frequently, action has to be formulated on the basis of a variety of evidence from differing sources. This may consist of several studies conducted by sundry investigators according to diverse designs and in various times and places. Rarely is such evidence wholly consistent and conclusive. In reviewing evidence from diverse sources, the following steps are helpful:

1. Discard studies which are irredeemably methodologically unsound. An understanding of the issues discussed in this book will help.
2. Try to quantify the likely magnitude and direction of any biases inherent to the remaining studies.
3. Where there are inconsistencies between studies, consider whether they might be due to any of the following:
   - subtle differences in aims and objectives;
   - different procedures (e.g. patient selection criteria and treatment regimens in a clinical trial);
   - lack of study power for the particular issue under consideration;
   - incidental secular trends between studies separated in time; or
   - differences in the underlying populations (biological, social and economic) of studies separated in space.

Informal meta-analysis entails using judgement, informed by the criteria above, to reach a plausible conclusion. It is sometimes helpful to see whether a panel of experts can reach consensus.

Formal meta-analysis entails a re-analysis of the original data from a series of studies of similar design. Each study is treated as if it were a component of one large new study. A single conclusion is reached for the aggregate. This process requires the construction of a statistical model (see pp. 177–8) encompassing all the studies. The model does not merely pool the data. It creates a structure which recognizes the features which differ between the studies. The technique has been used on a number of occasions in an attempt to form a conclusion from a series of individually inconclusive controlled trials.

Formal meta-analysis is coming into vogue but we have some reservations about its use:

1. The formal apparatus of statistical models can give a spurious sense of precision to an exercise which is strictly speaking comparing unlike things. By definition, the studies have not been designed to a common protocol or conducted under common quality control as in a true multi-centre study.
2. It is not clear that the tools of statistical inference, e.g. significance tests and confidence intervals, are valid in this context.
3. Assuming that the original studies were competently designed and had adequate statistical power, it follows that formal meta-analysis substitutes one large study for a series of smaller replicates. Independent replication of studies to confirm findings is a central method of science. Yet formal meta-analysis seeks to ignore this. It claims to be a procedure which overrides the necessarily informal assessment of whether a series of independently replicated studies bear out a common conclusion.
4. Formal meta-analysis may provide a seeming justification for weak studies which do not, and should not, stand up as evidence in their own right.

Examples of meta-analysis may be found in Goodman,[5] Gotzsche,[6] Libretti and Bertele[7] and Henderson *et al.*[8]

In conclusion, we are not saying that formal meta-analysis is wrong. However, beware those seeking to turn sows' ears into silk purses.

Chapter 12

Making evaluation work

Summary

This chapter links evaluation theory to NHS management practice. It identifies some salient concepts developed from decision theory including rational and non-rational choice. It is shown that there is much scope for optimism, particularly if the value of good information and good information skills are recognized.

The terrain

Evaluation is a rational process: from stated questions there is a logical sequence of steps which will yield an answer. The previous chapters have outlined this logic. It should by now be clear that sometimes there is a choice of possible routes to an answer; which route is selected will depend upon the circumstances of the evaluation, the investigator's underlying ideology and the resources available to the investigator. However, for each route there are objective criteria by which good and poor evaluative exercises may be distinguished. It may be that some authorities will quibble here and there about matters of emphasis in our development of the theme. Nevertheless, the territory of evaluation is broadly agreed and sufficiently well mapped to lead the traveller to safe ground. Unfortunately, when one leaves the technicalities of doing evaluation and moves to its use in decision making, there is no longer the comfort of a well-authenticated map. Moreover, such a map cannot exist as the topography of the terrain is for ever changing. We shall show that the traveller has moved into a region where the rational, the non-rational and the irrational compete. Even so, this is not cause for despair; there are guiding principles which, if used pragmatically, can dispel the cartographic nightmare.

Hitherto, in the context of the UK, the evaluation of health service effectiveness has been piecemeal, often of poor quality, and generally low on the management agenda. Perhaps the greatest criticism is that evaluations, and those who conduct them, are too often divorced from the decision-making machinery, e.g. how many health authorities have an expert in information science on their top management boards? Changes consequent upon the NHS and Community Care Act 1990 will, in our opinion, force evaluation high up the management agenda and bring about radical changes to information systems and decision making.

In essence, the NHS and Community Care Act 1990 separates the assessment of the health needs of populations and the purchase of services to meet those needs from the provision of services. The providers of services (e.g. hospitals) will compete for contracts from the purchasing arm of district health authorities. This creates several important opportunities for improving health service provision:

1. Services consumed need no longer be dictated by what happens to be provided. The purchasing teams will gradually be able to influence the provider units into structuring themselves to offer services dictated by the measured needs of populations.
2. Issues of service effectiveness and value for money will be considered by purchasing teams when exploring service provision options.
3. Quality of care, in its broadest sense, will be an issue in drawing up and monitoring contracts.

Thus the ethos of the health service will change radically. It will be necessary for managers to specify clear goals, aims and objectives, i.e. business plans. Detailed information on the cost and price of services will be demanded. Health care professionals will be forced to justify the effectiveness of their existing procedures. The introduction of innovation and alleged improvement will be subjected to greater scrutiny. Unfortunately, little present experience of health service decision making is readily applicable to the new NHS. Like it or not, managers and health care professionals will have to discard old ways of thinking and embrace the new. Evaluative modes of thinking and, in particular, the evaluation of service effectiveness, will become the norm rather than an optional extra as at present.

The issues being faced by the NHS in the UK apply to every health care system. The inescapable fact is that resources for health services are never likely to meet demand (demand by the public and demand by professionals for innovation) anywhere. Hence, inevitably there comes a point of crisis and structural changes are brought in to facilitate a more effective distribution of resources.

Decision making

In exploring the role of health service evaluation, it is useful to place it within the wider context of decision making and the supporting information systems. It is not our intention to advocate some grandiose theory of decision making. Nevertheless, it will be helpful to explore some of the insights which have emerged from thinkers in this area. We will then suggest a pragmatic approach. Many of the ideas discussed below have been taken from March[1] and applied to the health service. Reference to the original is strongly recommended.

Rationality: Some theories of choice

March[1] has stated that many theories of choice view decision making as rational and based on four things:

1. A *knowledge of alternatives*: this implies decision makers have a set of unambiguous alternatives to consider and act upon.
2. A *knowledge of consequences*: this assumes decision makers know the consequences of alternative actions (at least in probability terms).
3. A *consistent preference ordering*: that is, some objective means of ranking the subjective values attached to outcomes.
4. A *decision rule*: that is, a means of selecting a single course of action on the basis of its consequences for the preferences.

In these models of choice, it is often assumed that all pertinent information is known and that choice is made by selecting the option with the highest expected value.

Choice models of decision making are attractive and often helpful in understanding some decisions, e.g. the relationship between cost and demand. Moreover, March suggests that they are attractive within Western civilization because 'choice is a faith as well as a theory; it is linked to the ideologies of the Enlightenment'. This is manifested by the use of 'wilful choice' theories in many disciplines, e.g. economics, political science, psychology and sociology.

On this basis, senior health managers could therefore be exhorted to:

1. Determine clearly what their alternatives are.
2. Estimate the likely consequences stemming from each alternative and its chances of occurrence.
3. Define clearly what their preferences are.
4. Take the alternative which maximizes the expected value.

Planning guidance within the NHS has often been based on these premises, e.g. option analysis relating to decisions as to whether to build a new hospital or update an old one. However, in practice, the ideals listed cannot be met. To quote March:

> Theories of choice presume two improbably precise guesses about the future: a guess about the future consequences of current actions and a guess about future sentiments with respect to those consequences.

With regard to the first, lack of information is a restriction. Also, there are human computational problems, i.e. there are limits to the number of alternatives which can be held and manipulated. These ideas led Herbert Simon in the 1940s and 1950s to the notion of limited rationality – for which he won a Nobel prize in 1978. March summarizes this idea thus:

Rather than all alternatives or all information about consequences being known, information has to be discovered through *search*. *Search* is stimulated by a failure to achieve a goal, and continues until it reveals an alternative that is good enough to satisfy existing, evoked goals. New alternatives are sought in the neighbourhood of old ones. Failure focuses *search* on the problem of attaining goals that have been violated, success allows *search* resources to move to other domains. The key scarce resource is attention: and theories of limited rationality are, for the most part, theories of the allocation of attention.

The notion of not optimizing (choosing the best of all possible alternatives) but seeking a satisfactory solution is called *satisficing*.

Arising from the foregoing ideas is the notion of *slack*. When performance exceeds goals, *search* for new alternatives tends to be perfunctory, aspirations increase and *slack* accumulates. In contrast, when performance falls below goals, *search* is stimulated and *slack* and aspirations decrease. Thus *slack* is a store of unused *search* opportunities; it increases when goal attainment is easy and depletes when goal attainment is difficult.

These concepts are helpful in understanding the crisis management which tends to prevail in the NHS. For instance, they help explain why decision makers often appear to find new efficiencies during times of adversity; the reason being that during favourable times *slack* accumulates. It could be argued that the NHS, in its implementation of the NHS and Community Care Act 1990, is placing managers in an – initially – adverse environment and hence hoping to reduce *slack*. More energetic performance would be expected to occur during periods of adversity, but the price paid is that experiments in unusual techniques will be curtailed. These are more likely to occur in times of *slack*. This is contrary to the idea that necessity is the mother of invention.

Choice theories in recent times have thus paid attention to the fact that information gathering and processing place considerable demands on the choice makers. The uncertainty surrounding the future sentiments attached to current preferences poses difficulties. The assumptions made by choice theories are rigorous:

1. Preferences are absolute.
2. Preferences are stable.
3. Preferences are consistent and precise.
4. Preferences are not themselves affected by the choices proposed.

In practice, choices are often made without reference to fully conscious preferences. Also, March makes the point that human beings are aware that preferences are inconsistent and, as a result, engage in activities designed to manage preferences. They sometimes take action for no better reason that someone else is doing it so they must, i.e. they might shy away from choice decisions based on their preferences. As March stated: 'like Ulysses, they know the advantages of having their hands tied'.

Non-rationality: The politics of choice

Managers recognize that in reality preferences arise not wholly through rational argument or objective assessment of a situation. There are competing views and value systems. There is a process of argument and conflict. The selection of preferences can arise through consensus, compromise or domination. This is a political domain upon which simple and consistent rules of rationality cannot be imposed. This is an area of thought and action which we term *non-rational*. It is not irrational because each of the actors may be pursuing well-defined, but different, goals in a logical fashion. Yet, these goals may not be commensurate one with another. Hence no simple 'rational' rule may be explicated to guide decisions in these matters.

This issue may be made concrete by considering how choice might be made when purchasing health services for a defined population in the knowledge that resources are not available for every possibility. If this were to be approached wholly rationally, then the activity would have to be embedded in a generally agreed philosophy or ideology. There are several possibilities, including those listed in box 12.1.

Box 12.1   Examples of ideologies which could underlie the purchasing of health services

1. An approach to maximize the economic wealth of the nation. This implies concentrating resources on those who are economically active or soon to be economically active.
2. A Benthamite approach, i.e. utilitarianism. This would seek to maximize some health 'good' for the greatest number. Significant minorities might get short shrift.
3. A Marxist/Structuralist approach. This might concentrate on reducing differences in health experience between social groups, i.e. the so-called 'health inequalities'.
4. An equitable approach, i.e. fair shares for all. It is assumed that there is a working definition of fairness.
5. A self-interest approach. At governmental level, this might entail taking the course of action least likely to lose votes.

These approaches are philosophically incompatible. The problem is further compounded when preferences for courses of action to meet specific health needs are sought, e.g. reduction of ischaemic heart disease mortality. For instance, there is a trade-off in resources between long-term actions to prevent disease and short-term responses to ameliorate disease. This also implies a trade-off between the perceived loss through extant suffering and that through preventable suffering yet to occur.

Anyone who has ever sat on a health authority board or planning committee will know that an underlying ideology is rarely made explicit.

Furthermore, these groups do not hedge their bets by being Benthamites on Mondays and Marxists on Fridays. Indeed, it makes good sense not to be explicit for there never would be agreement. Hence, contrary to the expectations of rational theories of choice, it pays not to press these issues, for otherwise no diverse group of people would ever complete the first stage of decision making. In reality, preferences are formulated such as not to grossly dissatisfy each of the dominant members of the decision-making group.

The concept of *non-rationality* is helpful in understanding why other aspects of decision making diverge from the idealized world of rational choice. Choice theories underestimate the complexity and confusion which surrounds most decision making. Impinging on decision makers are the alliances of decision makers, the impact of changing technologies, the perceptions of the decision makers at the time and the attention individual decision makers are willing to devote to the problem. Individuals deal with a variety of problems. To some they give greater attention than to others. The attention given changes over time. Thus, the same problems can attract little or a lot of attention depending on other competing interests. Bearing this in mind, it is not surprising that decisions reached at one meeting are sometimes overturned at the next. A key person's attention may on the second occasion now be fixed on it, whereas at the previous meeting their attention had been fixed elsewhere. These considerations encompass what March calls *disorder*. This facet of decision making can be used under the heading 'if at first you don't succeed, try, try again'; the disorder phenomenon allows persistence to pay off.

Another *non-rational* influence explored by March is *symbolic action*. Choice theories assume that the primary reason for decision making is to make a choice. This may not be true – it may have a ritual or symbolic significance. Managers appear to spend little time in making decisions as compared to time spent meeting people and reviewing management performance. Formal decision making provides a ritual opportunity for allocating glory or blame, socializing, challenging or reconfirming power relationships, educating one's juniors and enjoying the pleasures of taking part in a choice decision. It is an arena in which symbolic actions take place.

In this drama, the audience needs to be assured of two things: first, the choice depends on rational, intelligent use of information and that constructive thinking and analysis has gone into it; secondly, the concerns of relevant people have been taken into account, i.e. the right people have been consulted prior to the decision. Organizational decision making is used to reinforce the idea that managers (and hence managerial decisions) affect an organization's performance. It is in this belief that performance-related pay depends.

This ritualistic aspect of decision making means outcomes are often of less importance than the process. In the NHS at the present moment, consumer satisfaction has a high priority. The decision process may therefore become one which shows the eagerness of management to accept and implement consumer proposals and symbolizes the dedication of the NHS staff to the principles of availability and service.

Information systems

The foregoing comments on decision making and choice have implications for the design of information systems for an organization. There are issues as to what information to gather and keep, to whom it should be provided and how to make it easily accessible and timely to those requiring it. There is also the question of cost and return. There are some general rules:

1. Don't buy information about something that cannot affect your choice.
2. Don't buy information if it will be freely available before a decision is required.
3. Don't buy information that confirms what you already know.

In fact, organizations do not follow these rules: they gather data and do not use them often, ask for more and then do not use them, make decisions and look for relevant information afterwards. There is some sense to what looks irrational. Decision makers tend to operate more in a surveillance role than in a problem-solving role.

They scan the organizational environment for surprises (e.g. NHS performance indicators) and take action according to rules (e.g. Department of Health and regional directives). Decision makers often sense that information is tainted. In theories of choice information is innocent. In reality, decision information is sometimes biased by the person or sub-group presenting it, e.g. by its selective use.

Decision makers are often subject to pressure from information givers and respected sources of good advice. It is not surprising that in some instances both might be ignored or one followed to the detriment of the other. It must be recognized that there is a symbolic element to information. As March states:

> Gathering and presenting information symbolizes (and demonstrates) the ability and legitimacy of decision makers. A good decision maker is one who makes decisions in a proper way, who exhibits expertise and uses generally accepted information. The competition for reputations among decision makers stimulates the over-production of information.

A case study

The following case study[2] illustrates some of the problems facing decision makers. The study arose when consultants in ophthalmology in a health district pressed for an additional consultant ophthalmologist to meet service needs. Comparative information was sought. Ophthalmology in the district had a lower length of stay and turnover interval than the regional average. It also had a higher throughput of cases. The district was compared in greater detail with two others. It was found that in the index district, the workload for whole-time equivalent consultants was greater than in the others. Also, there had over a period of 4 years been a 19% increase in new patients and a 28% increase in total out-patients. However, despite increased activity, waiting lists had risen. For one consultant, there was a waiting time of 75 weeks.

Before committing themselves to increasing the consultant establishment, the district management sought to explore the possibility of further improvements in efficiency. A 6-week work audit was performed with the consultants' consent. This revealed that one consultant spent only half his allocated theatre sessions actually in the operating theatre. Also, it was shown that cataract operations comprised 40% of total operations and that 14% of out-patient workload related to cataracts. In addition, there was a marked difference in workload between the three consultants.

A number of reasons were advanced as to why the problem occurred. These included:

1. Demographic changes: the elderly population of the district had increased.
2. Technical advances in cataract surgery led to increased pressure on services.
3. One consultant, without apparent reference to management, had changed a general clinic to a squint clinic. This caused a marked delay before the consultant saw cataract cases.

The decision makers went for the appointment of a new consultant, changing a 7-day ward to a 5-day ward and attempting to increase day surgery cases. They may have been swayed by factors other than those listed above: GPs complained through their local medical committee about lack of access of their patients, especially cataract patients; patients wrote to local newspapers complaining of delay; and the issue was taken up by local members of parliament.

It could be argued that the wrong decision was made. After all, there was evidence of differential work output between the three consultants and failure to fully utilize theatre sessions. In addition, the squint session could have been turned back into a general session.

This case study illustrates some of the points raised in relation to decision theory, e.g. decision makers' attention, the ritualistic use of information, an audit done but the results apparently ignored. These depressing circumstances raise the question of whether any formal attempts at evaluation are worth doing. Certainly, they will not be done well if those engaged on the task believe that their work is unlikely to influence decision making. In the next section, we explore how knowledge of the present dismal realities of health service decision making can be used to promote a more optimistic future.

Coping with uncertainty

William James[3], the great American Pragmatist, will be our guide through the land of the rational, the non-rational and the irrational. Pragmatism is a robust philosophy. It does not concern itself with a search for absolute truth. It accepts multiple 'truths' and can live with a measure of inconsistency among supposed 'truths'. It is directed by the 'cash-value' of ideas, i.e. their utility. Two quotations from James will suffice to give a flavour of pragmatism. On truth he writes:

Pragmatism, on the other hand, asks its usual question. 'Grant an idea or belief to be true,' it says, 'what concrete difference will its being true make to any one's actual life? How will the truth be realised? What experiences will be different from those which would obtain if the truth were false? What, in short, is the truth's cash-value in experiential terms?'

And on theory:

Theories thus become instruments, not answers to enigmas, in which we can rest. We don't lie back on them, we move forward, and on occasion, make nature over again with their aid.

It is apparent that the purpose of satisficing outlined on pp. 182–3 is in the spirit of pragmatism.

The practical problem facing decision makers is to maximize the rational, to eradicate the irrational and to live with the non-rational and, so far as possible, to reduce its scope (see Fig. 12.1).

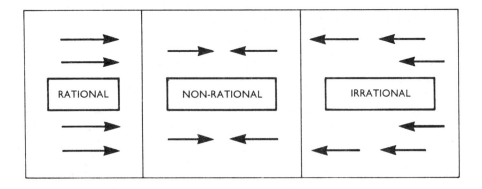

Fig. 12.1   Three modes of decision taking.

Handling the non-rational

The first step towards handling the non-rational is to accept its existence. The pragmatic decision maker will recognize that in the arena of the non-rational the laws of nature are those of politics (with a small 'p'). It is the domain of alliances of interests, brokerage of power, and subtle persuasion outside the formal meetings which ratify decisions. The key to this game is to identify the principal players. In this domain, it is legitimate to use information and evaluative exercises for their symbolic rather than factual content. The player who practises pragmatism and the teachings of Machiavelli[4] has an edge. He or she is not being unprincipled but merely playing by the unstated rules. Sadly, for some in the health service, the game appears to be an end in itself. Suspect the avid joiner of committees, the person for whom committee work is a joy rather than a necessary evil.

Nevertheless, the non-rational can be contained. This requires clearly stated procedures for consultation and decision making, and a determination by management not to allow itself to be deflected by players of wild cards once the procedures have properly been enacted. The pre-1991 NHS had elaborate procedures for consultation and decision making, yet too easily did management and the health authorities to whom they were answerable allow themselves to be swayed by minority pressure groups and vote-seeking politicians. This perhaps is forgivable as the pressure can be immense.

While the non-rational is ineradicable because it involves competing ideologies, it nevertheless can be prevented from being overwhelming if data about the local health service are made freely available in an intelligible and accessible form. Evaluation has a key role in this sharing of information.

The quality of public debate about health is poor. Misunderstanding mixed with powerful emotion and unattainable expectations may thwart attempts to reach reasonable solutions (cf. the case study on pp. 186–7). As the public is the paymaster for health services, they must ultimately receive what they are willing to pay for. However, the voices heard are those of representatives, self-styled and otherwise, and pressure groups – not those of the 'silent majority'. Clearly, before any particular ideology of self-interest is applied to health issues, it is desirable that certain incontestable factual information be shared. Thus, it is necessary for health service managers and service providers to become involved in dissemination of information to the public and its representatives.

Issues which sorely need to be understood include:

1. Health service funding must compete with funding for other public 'goods', e.g. education, roads, defence, the arts. More of one may mean less of another. All can grow only if the economy as a whole grows.
2. The level of public funding of health services may differ between governments, but it will never be enough to meet all existing demands or likely future demands.
3. Because funding will always be insufficient to meet demand, services must be rationed.
4. Rationing may be planned or occur by default. Waiting lists and the closure of hospital wards when funds run dry are examples of rationing by default. Planned rationing requires explicit choices between service options.
5. Services differ in their benefits for society as a whole and for individuals. Also, the benefit to one individual may implicitly deny benefit to others, e.g. one heart–lung transplant for cystic fibrosis may deny many hernia repairs or several hip-replacement operations. This is not to imply that heart–lung plumbers are interchangeable as hernia and hip repairmen. Rather, in funding the transplant service, there has been an opportunity cost with respect to hernias and hips. Rarely is opportunity cost explicitly recognized.
6. Formal techniques of evaluation can make explicit many of the issues

forming a rational starting point for the essentially non-rational process of choice, i.e. non-rationality need not be predicated upon irrationality.

The above must surely rank as incontrovertible, on a par with the laws of arithmetic. They set the context within which all ideological views on health must work.

Clearly, those non-rational aspects of decision making which take place within the health service, and which do not necessarily involve wider public debate, would also benefit if all the participants were better informed about the context in which choice is to be made. The education of managers and service providers will be discussed later.

Finally, there is a technique which is devastating within the rational and non-rational contexts. This is to be better prepared than others. Committees, which usually are the ultimate decision-making bodies, can be inherently incapable of being creative. This is so regardless of the talents of the individual members. In part, it is a consequence of their being dominated by local politics; Roberts[5] describes the NHS as a health care system 'run by politics'.

Thus, to present a committee with well-structured thoughts on an issue is half way to winning the argument. This ploy is particularly powerful if an ideological stance is not explicit and the case appears to rest solely on reasoning from authenticated factual material. A formal evaluation would constitute the background material. In this circumstance, the case can only be attacked on ideological grounds if others are willing to bring ideology forth but, as was suggested on pp. 184–5, it is usually in everyone's interests to fudge ideological matters. Thus, the mode of attack will be through weaknesses in the logic of the argument and inadequacies in the supporting material. Hence, a need to conduct sound evaluations for use in the domain of the non-rational. Conversely, anyone well versed in the theory of evaluation will be ideally placed to act as critic if an opponent plays this card.

Enhancing rationality

Critical modes of thought and an ability to conduct and/or understand evaluations are prerequisites for sensible planning within health services. In the introduction to this chapter, we suggested that the reforms to the NHS enacted in 1990 will encourage this. However, if the spirit of the Act is to be translated into action, local health service management will have to consider the structures within which planning takes place and the information sources feeding it.

Current information and planning systems may be criticized as follows. Information systems have tended to be formulated in isolation from the decision-making process. This has resulted in the *shopping list* principle, exemplified by the reports of the Korner Committee,[6] whereby information is to be gathered because it is believed to be useful, but there is little reference to how it should flow within the organization, be interpreted or inform decision making. Moreover, this opportunistic and atheoretical approach does not encourage systematic determination of information requirements and thereby tends towards that which is traditionally or readily available.

Planning procedures too often take place within a context of poorly explicated goals and aims and are constrained by existing information systems. Moreover, present 'planning' is conceptually incremental: it justifies the bolting on of additions, but does not question the basis for or value of what already exists – and is allowed to continue.

With regard to information systems, three points arise:

1. Evaluative work is much eased if high-quality and pertinent routine information is available.
2. Evaluation is a non-routine source of information.
3. It is possible to construct frameworks[7] for information requirements which avoid the 'shopping list' approach.

A central issue with respect to planning is that regardless of what, if any, theory drives decision making and regardless of rationality and non-rationality, the planning cycle has to be capable of encompassing evaluation. *Incremental planning* does not foster choice among alternative courses of action. Parallel planning does. *Parallel planning* demands that explicit choices be made.

Parallel planning occurs when new developments or other service changes have to compete simultaneously for funding within the context of some overall guiding principles. This is analogous to the manner in which research bodies distribute grants. All applications have to be received by a stated date and be presented in a standard format. Research applications are sifted first on the basis of their clarity and the soundness of the methods to be employed; often scoring systems are used. This sifting can be fairly objective as the scientific community is in reasonable agreement about what constitutes acceptable standards. The second stage is more likely to be in the domain of the non-rational. It entails judgement about the comparative scientific utility of a series of otherwise sound proposals.

Parallel planning should have occurred in the pre-reformation NHS: it is imperative in the new NHS. Purchasing groups will, after assessing the health needs of populations, be required to propose a package of services to be funded. These will include existing services and consideration of innovation. As there will be a fixed budget, choice will be mandatory. Moreover, the context will facilitate reappraisal of existing services and not merely the bolting on of the new. This is not going to be easy and the time-scale for major shifts in service emphasis will be a long one. Also, as a wide range of contracts will have to be negotiated at regular intervals, planning will perforce be parallel. Clearly, the impetus for this process will come from the purchasers. Nevertheless, the providers of services will not be passive sellers of their wares.

Providers will have to assess their long-term future. They will have to research the market for health care. They, being those most closely involved with day-to-day health care, will be in the best position to anticipate and try to sell technological advance. Like any good shopkeeper, they will make suggestions to the buyer about what he or she might care to purchase.

Hence, on both sides of the purchaser/provider divide, there will be a need for evaluation of options. The purchaser, however, is the one in the stronger position to state what criteria will be used in evaluation. This and related issues are discussed in a paper by St Leger *et al.*[8] Appendix B displays a checklist borrowed from the paper. It is designed to aid planners when assessing the merits of service options (particularly innovatory ones) during parallel planning. We suggest that a version of this to suit local circumstances should be used by both purchaser and provider.

Dispelling irrationality

Irrationality occurs within the service at two levels. The first occurs when the essentially rational elements of a planning process are allowed, through lack of managerial discipline, to be subverted. Unplanned, or so-called creeping, developments fall into this category. This was illustrated in the case study earlier (see pp. 186–7) when a consultant ophthalmologist had taken it upon himself to change a general out-patient clinic to squint clinic. Parallel planning and the exigencies of resourse management and clinical budgets should diminish this kind of abuse.

The second kind of irrationality is more complicated. It arises through key personnel being inappropriately trained, lacking confidence in their own critical faculties and being too easily swayed by forcefully expressed opinion rather than argument based on verifiable observation. It is in tackling this that the skills of evaluation, and the ethos of critical thinking that evaluation engenders, can help.

The training of the medical profession, certainly in the UK, may be at fault. Some of our supposedly most able young people – on the basis of school examination results – enter the profession. They are subjected to 5 or so years of heavily factually oriented training (not education). Claims that this training is scientific are questionable. It draws heavily on, sometimes transient, theory and factual insights from science, but it does not prepare a critical mind. On the contrary, it may be argued that the end result is to stultify the intellect and prepare an initiate to an hierarchical profession in which it is inadvisable to challenge 'authority'. Even at the higher reaches of the profession, there is tremendous peer pressure to conform and this is backed by subtle control through the merit award system.

Perhaps, the present programme of medical education and postgraduate training achieves its primary aim of producing safe doctors. However, few practitioners are fitted to the exigencies of the reformed NHS. If a critical ethos prevails, it will no longer be possible for practitioners to get their way by such utterances as:

This denies clinical freedom.

If you do (or do not) do this patients will suffer.

In my opinion as a practitioner of 30 years standing. . . .

To withhold this treatment from patients would be unethical.

It is not appropriate for us to prescribe detailed changes to the undergraduate curriculum. However, it is to be hoped that the General Medical Council, the Royal Colleges and their Faculties will realize that practitioners in the reformed NHS will not be effective advocates for the interests of their patients, and the wider population of potential patients, unless they take a serious interest in issues of health service planning. Clearly, there is a place for the inclusion of material on health care planning, management and evaluation within postgraduate training programmes of all specialities.

Lest we be misunderstood, we are not with respect to evaluation advocating that every doctor be required at some stage in their training to gain considerable research skills and engage in research or evaluation. On the contrary, it would be better if fewer were under pressure to produce a scatter of inconsequential published papers to impress appointments committees. Nevertheless, every practitioner ought to be able to read, critically, published research in their field and to be able to apply a checklist such as that in Appendix B sensibly. Indeed, medical audit is a major feature of the NHS reform. It will require every clinician, eventually, to be able to define objectives against which the service can be evaluated; it will also require the development of interpersonal skills so that the lessons from audit can be applied positively and constructively to patient care, and not to witch hunt or destroy unfortunate individuals. And similar remarks apply in varying degree to nursing and the other paramedical disciplines.

It is to management that we look for the main impetus towards critical thinking. Management must gain confidence to question medical opinion more thoroughly; the checklist provides the framework for this. Lay managers must appreciate that 5 or more years of medical training is not necessary to give competence or authority to ask pertinent and searching questions, and to demand answers backed by evidence. It would be beneficial if management training programmes were reviewed with this in mind. Also, management may look to public health medicine as a bridge between themselves and clinical practice. Indeed, it is desirable that management trainees and public health trainees be taught alongside each other for part of their respective training programmes.

Resources for evaluation

In the UK, and in varying degrees elsewhere, research and development in health care and evaluation are poorly resourced and badly organized locally and nationally. In comparison to major industries, the NHS allocation towards research and development is pitifully small.

It is perhaps not reasonable for the NHS to support fundamental research in the biomedical sciences; this is better left to the research councils, charities and pharmaceutical industry. However, end-stage ('near market') development and evaluation of innovation should be in the NHS remit. Only thus will evaluation be done according to criteria which meet the information requirements of NHS planners.

The evaluation of major developments is too large a task for individual health authorities. Moreover, in order that effort be not duplicated and that common standards apply, it requires national co-ordination. This is important not least because large-scale evaluation is expensive and the choice of what is to be evaluated should be guided by some explicit priorities. Patel *et al.*[9] suggest how such co-ordinated effort might be effected.

At district level, in provider units, purchasing bodies and Family Health Services Authorities, there is need to reappraise the funding of information services and evaluation. However, there is a serious obstacle. This is the specious notion that money should not be diverted from 'direct patient care'. This first cousin of shroud waving has too often prevented the development of management systems. The fact is that money will always be tight. There will be an opportunity cost of money diverted from direct patient care. However, that opportunity cost in terms of patient outcome cannot be known because so little of what is done in the name of direct patient care is of proven effectiveness or efficiency. The diversion of funds will provide the basis for answering questions about effectiveness and efficiency.

The problem with information systems at present is that they tend to be badly thought out (see pp. 190–2) and poorly led. The latter is hardly surprising as information management is seen as a back room technician's job. There is no clearly defined career structure within information services in the NHS. Staff tend to wander in and out of information on their upward path to better things. It is time that information officers were put on a par with other professional groupings in the NHS. Perhaps, information officers and information managers should be on the scientific officer scale which culminates at a very senior level. In conjunction with the universities and polytechnics, training programmes should be formulated for this profession. An appropriate training would include epidemiology. The essential skills of these people will be the interpretation of information; the running of computers *can* be left to technicians. Moreover, a more radical approach would be to link information services with traditional library services.

If, as we believe, information will be central to the proper functioning of the reformed NHS, then at least one member of the top management board of each provider unit, purchaser and FHSA should be well versed in the discipline.

Although all senior managers, clinicians and paramedicals should be versed in evaluation lore, there is still a need for more specialist expertise to direct particular evaluative exercises and for support staff for those exercises. In some cases, money might best be spent on in-house staff, in others expertise might be bought from outside, e.g. university departments of public health. The cost of in-house support staff (e.g. survey teams), may be reduced by drafting trainees from a variety of disciplines *including management.* In addition, one of the most valuable sources of help is a research nurse. These nurses, with appropriate training and experience, cannot only provide leadership to survey teams but also engender trust and respect in clinical settings.

Summing up

The central theme of this chapter has been that health service evaluation can only be of benefit if it takes place within a structure which demands and can use the kind of information that evaluation provides. The reforms to the NHS offer the opportunity for more thoughtful and effective management which will be of benefit to patients. The opportunity can be realized only if management grasp the nettle of disciplined decision making and proper funding of support services. It should not be assumed that other professional groups within the NHS will perceive this to be to their advantage. Thus to get the edge, management must become effective in applying critical thought to clinical practice. They must call upon help from wherever they can find it.

We conclude by quoting the closing paragraph from Cochrane's *Effectiveness and Efficiency* (see Further reading list) and leave our readers to make up their minds whether a rational health service has yet been gained:

> My colleagues, in their devotion to their patients, evoke my admiration, but also remind me of Agatha in Eliot's 'The Family Reunion', who wanted action:
>
>> Not for the good it will do
>> But that nothing may be left undone
>> On the margin of the impossible
>
> I hope clinicians in the future will abandon the pursuit of the 'margin of the impossible' and settle for 'reasonable probability'. There is a whole rational health service to gain.

Appendix A

Obtaining data

Introduction

This appendix is divided into four main sections as follows: demographic data; activity data; health and disease data; and information services. The material is structured by taking subjects on which data are required and then listing the sources (see Table 4.6) where the data can be found, rather than by taking sources of data and listing what data are available from each source. This is rather clumsy when dealing with large sources of data, such as the census, but overall it facilitates finding data on a given subject.

Demographic data

Population data

The baseline population data, from which all other population data are derived, are the results of the 1981 census. The district population and the age breakdown is contained in an OPCS booklet called *Census 1981: Key Statistics for Local Authorities*. 1991 census details will be available from OPCS.

The Longitudinal Study User Manual is obtainable from SSRU, City University, Northampton Square, London EC1V 0HB, UK.

Population estimates and projections

Population estimates refer to educated guesses of the population from the time of the last census to the present day, while population projections refer to educated guesses of the population in the future. Population estimates are calculated by OPCS by taking the census data as a baseline, by using data on births and deaths since the time of the census, and then estimating migration in and out of the district. The address for OPCS is: OPCS, Tichfield, Fareham, Hants PO15 5RR, UK.

Births

The Director of Public Health should be notified of all births in the district within 36 hours. Fertility rates and total births are available by legitimacy, birth weight and social class from OPCS.

Social characteristics

Most of the information available on the social characteristics of the people comes from the census. The book *Census 1981: Key Statistics for Local Authorities*, contains the following information for districts. Similar details will be available from the 1991 census.

- economic activity;
- industry of employment (10% sample);
- travel to work (10% sample);
- number of households/household size/economically active adults; and
- households with children/one-adult households with children.

Note that country of birth is available from previous censuses but was not recorded in 1991. Thus, this book contains most of the data on social indicators which are available from the census.

As regards electoral ward data, the following information may be obtained from a regional health authority or from a local authority:

- % of the population of at least 65 years of age;
- % of elderly people living alone;
- % of the population under 5 years of age;
- % of families that are one-parent families;
- % of the workforce who are unskilled;
- % of the workforce who are unemployed;
- % of households that lack basic amenities; and
- % of the population who were born in countries other than the UK.

For an overall score for the ward regarding indices of social deprivation, see Jarman, B. (1983). Identification of underprivileged areas. *British Medical Journal*, **286**: 1705–8; Townsend, P., Phillimore P. and Beattie, A. (1986). *Inequalities in Health in the Northern Region: An Interim Report*. Northern Regional Health Authority, Bristol.

Activity data

Hospital information (including day cases and out-patients)

The information systems at present collecting hospital information are (1) Hospital Management Information System (HMIS: Korner Aggregated Returns) and (2) performance indicators.

Hospital Activity Analysis (HAA) became Korner statistics in April 1987, and included some information on psychiatric and maternity patients. It was introduced in 1969 by the DHSS and was a summary of the case notes of all patients discharged from non-mental hospitals. The information was collected by medical records departments and collated regionally.

HAA was a computerized system for recording all in-patient and day case activity other than maternity and psychiatry. The coding form illustrates the large variety of information available from the system, e.g. main and other diagnoses, main and other operations, area of residence, age, sex, consultant, source of admission, disposal and length of time on the waiting list. A 10% sample of information was submitted by regional health authorities to OPCS. This formed the basis of the Hospital In-patient Enquiry (HIPE) tables published annually. HIPE ceased at the end of 1986.

Information could be obtained from HAA on length of stay, age on admission, disposal on discharge, source of admission and cases admitted from the waiting list. In addition, there was information on diagnosis (coded according to the International Classification of Diseases), type of operation and total length of hospital stay.

An HAA system for maternity was available. Information for the remaining speciality excluded from the HAA system, namely psychiatry, was recorded on the Mental Health Enquiry System (see below).

The Hospital Management Information System (HMIS), now called Korner Aggregated Returns System (KARS), is an administrative system. It records activity but does not record either diagnoses or procedures carried out. VS forms are derived from this system. It is usually recorded more completely than HAA data. It is usually processed by regional health authorities.

The Mental Health Enquiry (MHE) system recorded information about psychiatric patients discharged from hospital. The data were sent to the DHSS at Fleetwood where they were transferred to a computer. The MHE ceased in 1986; it was replaced in April 1987 by a system similar to HAA.

Performance indicators: the term 'performance indicators' can mean many things, but the performance indicators which are routinely available are mainly concerned with activity rather than with outcome, and so are of limited use as an epidemiological tool. There are two packages of performance indicators available, produced by (a) the DHSS and (b) the Health Services Management Centre in Birmingham. The discs run on the BBC microcomputer and also on IBM compatible machines. Information on DHSS performance indicators can be obtained from the DHSS: contact DHSS, Room 1418, Euston Tower, 286 Euston Road, London NW1 3DN, UK.

No diagnostic information is routinely recorded on day hospital patients or out-patients.

Health service activity in the community

General Practitioners

Until recently, little routine information was available on the activity of GPs. However, in the future, GP annual reports to the FHSA should be a valuable source of information. At present, the FHSA should know the total number of prescriptions written by all GPs and, for 1 month of the year, the number of prescriptions written by each GP.

Services to the community

These include:

- vaccination and immunization, obtainable from Korner statistics;
- family planning services, obtainable from Korner statistics;
- school health services, obtainable from form 8MI; and
- maternity and child health services, obtainable from Korner statistics.

Health and disease data

This section is divided into four parts as follows: mortality data, morbidity data, health status and health outcome.

Mortality data

A copy of the death registration of every resident who dies in the district or elsewhere is sent to the Director of Public Health Medicine. District mortality data are processed by OPCS and are available as VS returns. They contain some details of the number of people who died in the district from a large number of conditions (using the ICD code). The data are presented by age and sex.

OPCS 'death tapes' at district level

OPCS provides 'death tapes' to regions. Before 1981, data did not include ward and postcode; subsequently, they have been included. It is now possible to build up a map of deaths by ward for a district from these tapes. Analysis can be aided by using a computer program to interrogate the database.

FIND is a computer program developed by Dr Whitten of the School of Environmental Science at the University of Bradford for this purpose. The selection criteria include: particulars of registration, sex, cause of death, particulars of occupation, place of birth, date of birth, date of death, postcode and ward.

Morbidity data

Infectious diseases

Episodes of notifiable infectious diseases are reported to the Local Authority Proper Office, who is usually a consultant in public health medicine. The Communicable Disease Surveillance Centre (CDSC) produces the Communicable Disease Report (CDR) weekly. The CDR lists the number of cases of the more common infectious diseases, which have been diagnosed in public health laboratories around the country. It also contains reports on interesting outbreaks and cases of infectious diseases.

Prescribable diseases

Data on the number of prescribable (occupational certifiable) diseases are available from the Health and Safety Executive.

Neoplastic diseases

Incidence data on patients with malignant neoplasms (and a few benign neoplasms) are compiled by the Cancer Registry.

Incidence of diseases in the community

There is no routine system of measuring disease incidence in the community. Korner collects information on the diagnoses of people who are admitted to hospital, but in most conditions the number of hospital admissions for a condition is a poor measure of its incidence in the community, partly because not everyone with a given disease will be treated in hospital, and partly because Korner reflects events rather than patients.

Health status

Ideally, information should be available on the health status of your district. To obtain this, a local survey is usually necessary. An example is the health survey of Stockport

Health Authority residents, which was based on a random sample of 1:100 Stockport residents.

Health outcome

This can be measured in a number of ways, e.g. the mortality or morbidity resulting from a procedure, or by looking at the effect of a procedure on the quality of life. From the district point of view, mortality data are the easiest to obtain; death certificates of every resident who dies in the district, or elsewhere, are sent to the Director of Public Health. Morbidity is more difficult, and a local survey may be necessary. The Royal College of General Practice have published data on morbidity in general practice. The Nottingham Health Profile has been used to assess improvements in the quality of life following procedures.

Information services

In *Providing a District Library Service* (Kings Fund, London, 1985) the following statement is made:

> Staff dealing with emergencies require information quickly. For currency, accuracy and speed of access an on-line data base will usually provide the most appropriate form of service. Useful national resources could include: poisons information, drug information, infectious disease trends, and blood products and transplant data. Local databanks might cover hospital resources, major accident procedures and laboratory investigation requirements. Often the information would be accessed directly by a clinician rather than through a librarian for reasons of speed or confidentiality. In some cases the library terminal will be used to provide access to these databanks. The librarian should contribute to training in the use of on-line systems and advice on choice of equipment.

These needs can be met using a BBC or IBM compatible microcomputer plus printer and a modem with access to Data Star Base. There is special NHS rate for using Data Star.
  A suitable format is as follows:

1. Joint Packet switch stream British Telecom Network
   Address: Customer Service Department
             20th Floor, St Andrew's House
             Portland Street, Manchester M1 3LH, UK.
2. Suitable modem: Pace Nightingale Comm. Star Combination
   Address: Pace Micro Technology
             Juniper View
             Allerton Road
             Bradford, West Yorkshire, UK

Join Data Star is a computerized information service. Databases available include DHSS database, Biomedical databases, e.g. Medline and Management Contents database.

Costs: There is a standard charge plus charge depending on usage. Alternatively, obtain access to a library which has an on-line computer linked into databases and pay a fee per search.

Appendix B

Template for a checklist for the evaluation of innovatory proposals

1. Describe clearly and concisely the proposal, indicating how its development differs from and is likely to enhance current practice. (What does it do, to whom, how, why etc.?)
2. What, in detail, is the proposal intended to achieve?
   (a) Beneficiaries – group number, etc.
   (b) Demand
      - INITIAL – numbers, cost
      - FINAL – numbers, cost – containment of demand?
   (c) Benefits – projected outcome
      - quantification
      - monitoring
      - assessment
        — change in life expectancy
        — quality of life
        — morbidity, etc.
   (d) Problems/hazards
3. What, in detail, are the projected costs of the proposal?
   (a) Any initial capital costs
   (b) Staffing implication
   (c) Anticipated marginal costs invoked on expansion
   (d) If demand exceeds this present proposal, what is the upper limit at which increased capital and manpower costs would occur?
   (e) Will other developments be lost or deferred or altered if this proposal is adopted?
   (f) Will any savings accrue?
4. What is the evidence that the proposal will provide benefit?
   (a) Preliminary formal trial   (Yes/No)
      - Was it randomized?   (Yes/No)
        If not, why not?   ....
      - Were the following aspects adequate?
        DESIGN, SIZE, CONDUCT, ANALYSIS, INTERPRETATION
      - Was cost-effectiveness or cost–benefit assessed?
      - Were the criteria of COST, BENEFIT and EFFECTIVENESS appropriate to the presently envisaged realization of the service?

- Do the findings of the trial (a) justify the assertions under (2) above and (b) can they be extrapolated to the kind of populations for whom this service is intended?
- If there have been several separate trials, are the findings reproducible and consistent? (Yes/No)
  If not, how do the results affect the answers given under (2) above?
(b) Experience of implementation elsewhere
  - Has the proposed innovation been practised elsewhere?
  - Is there previously published, or otherwise accessible, work?
  - What has been learned from this experience?
  - What changes, if any, would be recommended for the present proposal?
  - Was the demand for this practice contained?
  - What costs were involved?
  - Were the benefits consistent with those suggested under (2) above?
(c) If the answers to (a) and (b) are negative or equivocal:
  - Should a formal study or trial be considered?
  - Where should the study be done?
  - How would such a study be funded?
  - Should a decision on implementation be deferred until other people's findings are known?
5. Are other developments, e.g. alternative methods of treatment or care, likely to overtake the current proposal?
   Should these be considered before any implementation?
6. If the proposal is adopted, how is it to be evaluated for:
   (a) Outcome
   (b) Cost-effectiveness
   (c) Performance – relating to targets for continuation of expenditure?
   If the service is being introduced on a pilot basis, have criteria been agreed for the circumstances in which ultimately the service might be withdrawn?

Source: St Leger, A.S., Allen, D. and Rowsell, K.V. (1989). Procedures for the evaluation of innovatory proposals. *British Medical Journal*, **299**: 1017–18. (Reproduced with the permission of the Editor).

References

Chapter 1: An overview of evaluation
1. Fowler, H.W. and Fowler, F.G. (1934). *The Concise Oxford Dictionary of Current English*. Oxford University Press, Oxford.
2. Donabedian, A. (1980). *Explorations in Quality Assessment and Monitoring. Vol. 1: The Definition of Quality and Approaches to its Assessment*. Health Administration Press, Ann Arbor, Mich.
3. *World Health Organization (1989). Quality Assurance in Health Care*, Vol. 1, No. 2/3. WHO, Geneva.
4. Various authors (1989). Rapid epidemiological assessment. *International Journal of Epidemiology*, **18** (suppl. 12).

Chapter 2: Key concepts and the setting of objectives
1. Maxwell, R.J. (1984). Quality assessment in health. *British Medical Journal*, **288**: 1470-1.

Chapter 4: Using routinely gathered data to assist in evaluation
1. The source of this excellent idea eludes us. It is thoroughly integrated into our thinking yet, sadly, we are unable to give due credit to its originator.
2. Rhind, D. (ed.) (1983). *A Census User's Handbook*. Methuen, London.
3. Talbot, R.J. (1991). Underprivileged areas and health care planning: implications of use of Jarman indicators of urban deprivation. *British Medical Journal*, **302**: 383-6.
4. Smith, G.D. (1991). Second thoughts on the Jarman index. *British Medical Journal*, **302**: 359-60.
5. Office of Population, Census and Surveys (1985). *William Far 1807-1883: Commemorative Symposium*. Occasional Paper 33. HMSO, London.
6. *Morbidity Statistics from General Practice - Third National Study* (1986). HMSO, London.
7. *Morbidity Statistics from General Practice - Third National Study, Socio-economic Analyses* (1990). HMSO, London.
8. Read, J.D. (1990). Computerising medical language. *British Journal of Health Care Computing, Conference Proceedings*, HC90: 203-8.
9. Department of Health and Social Security (1982). *Steering Group on Health Services Information 1st Report to the Secretary of State* (the Korner Report). HMSO, London.

10. Bardsley, M., Cole, J. and Jenkins, L. (eds) (1987). *DRGs and Health Care: The Management of Case Mix*. Oxford University Press, Oxford.
11. British Medical Association (1989). *An Evaluation of the Six Experimental Sites by the Central Consultants and Specialists Committee of the British Medical Association*. Resource management initiative. BMA, London.
12. Hornbrook, M.C. (1982) Hospital case mix: its definition, measurement and use. *Part 1: The conceptual framework; Part 2: Review of alternative measures. Medical Care Review*, **39**: 1–43, 73–123.

Chapter 5: Some basic economic concepts and their uses
1. Kind, P., Rosser, R. and Williams, A. (1982). Valuation of the quality of life: Some psychometric evidence. In M.W. Jones Lee (ed.), *The Value of Life and Safety*. North-Holland, Amsterdam, pp. 159–70.
2. Fallowfield, L. (1990). *The Quality of Life: The Missing Measurement*. Souvenir Press, London.
3. Williams, A. (1985). Economics of coronary artery bypass grafting. *British Medical Journal*, **291**, 326–9.

Chapter 6: Descriptive, testimony, case studies and case-control studies
1. Social Services Inspectorate (1986). *Inspection of the Supervision of Social Workers in the Assessment and Monitoring of Cases of Child Abuse, when Children Subject to a Court Order, have been Returned Home*. HMSO, London.
2. Department of Health and Social Security (1988). *Protecting Children: A Guide for Social Workers*. HMSO, London.
3. Chinese Health Information Centre Evaluation Subgroup of Steering Committee (1989). *Chinese Health Information Centre Evaluation 1987-9*. CHIC, Manchester.
4. Welton, R. and Barker, P. (1989). *Service Effectiveness Report: Day Case Surgery Preston* (Officers Report). Preston Health Authority, Preston.
5. Boyle, M.E., Pitts, M.K., Phillips K.C. *et al.* (1989). Exploring young people's attitudes to and knowledge of Aids: The value of focused group discussion. *Health Education Journal*, **48** (1): 21–3.
6. NHS Training Authority (1987). *Templeton Series on District General Managers*. NHS Training Authority, Gloucestershire.
7. Brown, R.M.A. and Perkins, M.J. (1989). Child sexual abuse presenting as organic disease. *British Medical Journal*, **299**: 614–15.
8. Kane, N.M. and Manoukian, P.D. (1989). The effect of the Medicare prospective payment system on the adoption of new technology. *New England Journal of Medicine*, **321**: 1378–83.
9. Stocking, B. (1985) *Initiative and Inertia: Case Studies in the NHS*. Nuffield Provincial Hospitals Trust, London.
10. Frankel, S., Farrow, A. and West, R. (1989). Non-admission or non-invitation? A case-control study of failed admissions. *British Medical Journal*, **299**: 598–600.
11. MacDonald, N.J., McConnell, K.N., Stephen, M.R. *et al.* (1989). Hypernatraemic dehydration in patients in a large hospital for the mentally handicapped. *British Medical Journal*, **299**: 1426–9.
12. Thompson, R.S., Rivara, F.P. and Thompson, D.C. (1989). A case-control study of the effectiveness of bicycle helmets. *New England Journal of Medicine*, **320**: 1361–7.

Chapter 7: Intervention studies
1. Black, N. (1985). Glue ear: the new dyslexia? *British Medical Journal*, **290**: 163–5.

2. Maran, A.G.D. and Wilson, J.A. (1986). Glue ear and speech development. *British Medical Journal*, **293**: 713.
3. Smithells, R.W., Sheppard, S. and Schorah, C.J. (1976) Vitamin deficiencies and neural type defects. *Archives of Diseases of Childhood*, **51**: 944–50.
4. Smithells, R.W., Sheppard, S., Schorah, C.J. *et al.* (1980). Possible prevention of neural-tube defects by periconceptual vitamin supplementation. *Lancet*, **1**: 339–40.
5. Pocock, S.J. (1987). *Clinical Trials: A Practical Approach*. John Wiley, Chichester.
6. Cochrane, A.L. (1972). *Effectiveness and Efficiency: Random Reflections on Health Services*. Nuffield Provincial Hospitals Trust, London.
7. Thompson, D.R. (1989). A randomized controlled trial of in-hospital nursing support for first time myocardial infarction patients and their partners: Effects on anxiety and depression. *Journal of Advanced Nursing*, **14**: 291–7.
8. Benson, D.W., Griggs, B.A., Hamilton, F. *et al.* (1990). Clogging of feeding tubes: A randomized trial of a newly designed tube. *Nutritional Clinical Practice*, **5**: 107–10.
9. Roe, B.H. (1990). Study of the effects of education on the management of urine drainage systems by patients and carers. *Journal of Advanced Nursing*, **15**: 517–24.
10. Rush, J., Fiorino-Chiovitti, R., Kaufman, K. *et al.* (1990). A randomized controlled trial of a nursery ritual: Wearing cover gowns to care for healthy newborns. *Birth*, **17**: 25–30.
11. Conine, T.A., Daechsel, D., Choi, A.K. *et al.* (1990). Costs and acceptability of two special overlays for the prevention of pressure sores. *Rehabilitative Nursing*, **15**: 133–7.
12. Gribbin, M. (1981). Placebos: Cheapest medicine in the world. *New Scientist*, **89**: 64–5.
13. Medical Research Council Working Party (1977). Randomized controlled trial of treatment for mild hypertension: Design and pilot trial. *British Medical Journal*, **1**: 1437–40.
14. Medical Research Council Working Party (1985). MRC trial of treatment of mild hypertension: Principal results. *British Medical Journal*, **291**: 97–104.
15. Diabetic Retinopathy Research Group (1976). Preliminary reports on effects of photocoagulation therapy. *American Journal of Ophthalmology*, **81**: 383–96.
16. James, I.M., Griffith, D.N.W., Pearson, R.M. *et al.* (1980). Effect of oxprenolol on stage-fright in musicians. *Lancet*, **2**: 952–4.
17. Cochran, W.G. and Cox, G.M. (1957). *Experimental Designs*. John Wiley, New York.
18. Canadian Cooperative Study Group (1978). A randomized trial of aspirin and sulfinpyrazone in threatened stroke. *New England Journal of Medicine*, **299**: 53–9.
19. Peto, R., Pike, M.C., Armitage, P. *et al.* (1976). Design and analysis of randomized clinical trials requiring prolonged observation of each patient: I. Introduction and design. *British Journal of Cancer*, **34**: 585–612.
20. Peto, R., Pike, M.C., Armitage, P. *et al.* (1977). Design and analysis of randomized clinical trials requiring prolonged observation of each patient: II. Analysis and examples. *British Journal of Cancer*, **35**: 1–39.
21. Johnstone, E.C., Deakin, J.F.W., Lawler, P. *et al.* (1980). The Northwick Park electroconvulsive therapy trial. *Lancet*, **2**: 1317–20.
22. Petch, M.C. (1983). Coronary bypasses. *British Medical Journal*, **287**: 514–16.
23. Hampton, J.R. (1984). Coronary artery bypass grafting for the reduction of mortality: An analysis of the trials. *British Medical Journal*, **289**: 1166–70.
24. McDowell, I. and Newell, C. (1987). *Measuring Health: A Guide to Rating Scales and Questionnaires*. Oxford University Press, Oxford.

25. Gehan, E.A. and Freireich, E.J. (1974). Non-randomized controls in cancer clinical trials. *New England Journal of Medicine*, 290: 198–203.
26. Cranberg, L. (1979). Do retrospective controls make clinical trials 'inherently' fallacious? *British Medical Journal*, 2: 1265–6.
27. Sacks, H., Chalmers, T.C. and Smith, H. (1982). Randomized versus historical controls for clinical trials. *American Journal of Medicine*, 72: 233–40.
28. Diehl, L. and Perry, D.J. (1986). A comparison of randomized concurrent control groups with matched historical controls: Are historical controls valid? *Journal of Clinical Oncology*, 4: 114–20.
29. Jennet, B. (1983) *High Technology Medicine: Benefits and Burdens*. The Nuffield Provincial Hospitals Trust, London.
30. Temple, R. (1990). Problems in the use of large data sets to assess effectiveness. *International Journal of Technology Assessment in Health Care*, 6: 211–19.
31. Jackson, R.P.J. (1985). The evaluation of clinical trials. *Postgraduate Medical Journal*, 61: 133–9.
32. Thomas, H.F., Elwood, P.C., Welsby, E. *et al.* (1979). Relationship of blood lead in women and children to domestic water lead. *Nature*, 282: 712–13.

Chapter 8: Assessing patient satisfaction

1. Department of Health and Social Security (1983). *National Health Service Management Inquiry* (Griffith Report). London.
2. Reid, M.E. and McIlwaine, G.M. (1980). Consumer opinion of a hospital antenatal clinic. *Social Science and Medicine*, 14A: 363–8.
3. Burnley, Pendle and Rossendale Community Health Council (1983). *Barnoldswick Survey: Report on Public Opinion*. Burnley.
4. Cartwright, A. and Anderson, R. (1981). *General Practice Revisited*. Tavistock/Methuen, London.
5. Kings Fund (1977). *Patients and Their Hospitals*. Kings Fund, London.
6. Hurst, K. (1986). *Patients' Expectations of and Satisfaction with Their Nursing Care*. Report No. 3, Central Nottinghamshire Health Authority, Nursing Research Section.
7. Ho Siew Fern and Scott, M. (1988). *A Report on North Manchester General Hospital Out-patient Survey*. North Western Regional Health Authority, Manchester.
8. Kerruish, A., Wickens, I. and Tarrant, P. (1988). Information from patients as a management tool: Empowering managers to improve the quality of care. *Hospital and Health Services Review*, April: 64–7.
9. Trent, H. (1981). What the public wants. *Health and Social Service Journal*, 5 June: 665–8.

Chapter 9: The evaluation of disease prevention services

1. Green, L.W. and Anderson, C.L. (1986). *Community Health*. Times Mirror/Mosby College Publishing, St Louis.
2. Puska, P., Tuomilehto, J., Salonen, J. *et al.* (1979). Changes in coronary artery risk factors during a comprehensive five year community programme to control cardiovascular diseases. *British Medical Journal*, 2: 1173–8.
3. Salonen, J.T., Puska, P. and Mustaniemi, H. (1979). Changes in morbidity and mortality during comprehensive community programme to control cardiovascular diseases during 1972–7 in North Karelia. *British Medical Journal*, 2: 1178–83.
4. Wilson, J.M.G. and Jungner, G. (1968). *Principles and Practice of Screening for Disease*. WHO Public Health Paper No. 34. WHO, Geneva.

5. Shapiro, S., Venet, W., Strax, P. *et al.* (1982). Ten- to fourteen-year effect of breast cancer screening on mortality. *Journal of the National Cancer Institute*, **69**: 349-55.
6. Verbeek, A.L.M., Hendricks, J.H.C.L., Holland, R. *et al.* (1984). Reduction of breast cancer mortality through mass screening with modern mammography: First results of the Nijmegen Project, 1975-1981. *Lancet*, 1: 1222-4.
7. Colette, H.J.A., Day, N.E., Rombach, J.J. *et al.* (1984). Evaluation of screening for breast cancer in a non-randomized study (the DOM project) by means of a case control study. *Lancet*, 1: 1224-6.
8. Tabar, L., Gad, A., Holmberg, L.H. *et al.* (1985). Reduction in mortality from breast cancer after mass screening with mammography. *Lancet*, 1: 829-32.
9. Department of Health and Social Security (1986). *Breast Cancer Screening* (the Forrest Report). HMSO, London.
10. Roberts, M., Alexander, F.E., Anderson, T.J. *et al.* (1990). Edinburgh trial of screening for breast cancer: Mortality at seven years. *Lancet*, 1: 241-6.
11. Day, N.E., Baines, C.J., Chamberlain, J. *et al.* (1986). UICC project on screening for cancer: Report of workshop on screening for breast cancer. *International Journal of Cancer*, 38: 303-8.
12. Baines, C.J. (1987). Breast cancer screening: Current evidence on mammography and implications for practice. *Canadian Family Physician*, 33: 915-21.
13. Veterans Administration Cooperative Study Group on Anti-hypertensive Agents (1970). Effects of treatment on morbidity in hypertension, II. Results in patients with diastolic blood pressure averaging 90 through 114 mmHg. *Journal of the American Medical Association*, **213**: 1143-52.
14. US Public Service Hospitals Cooperative Study Group (1977). Treatment of mild hypertension: Results of a ten year intervention trial. *Circulation Research*, I: 98-105 (suppl.).
15. Report by the Management Committee (1980). The Australian therapeutic trial in mild hypertension. *Lancet*, 1: 1261-7.
16. Helgeland, A. (1980). The Oslo study, treatment of mild hypertension: A five year controlled drug trial. *American Journal of Medicine*, **69**: 725-32.
17. Medical Research Council Working Party (1985). MRC trial of treatment of mild hypertension: Principal results. *British Medical Journal*, **291**: 97-104.
18. Amery, A., Birkenhager, W., Brixko, P. *et al.* (1985). Mortality and morbidity results from the European Working Party on high blood pressure in the elderly trial. *Lancet*, 1: 1349-54.
19. Garraway, W.M., Akhtar, A.J., Prescott, R.J. *et al.* (1980). Management of acute stroke in the elderly: Preliminary results of a controlled trial. *British Medical Journal*, **280**: 1040-3.
20. Garraway, W.M., Akhtar, A.J., Hockey, L. *et al.* (1981). Management of acute stroke in the elderly: Follow up of a controlled trial. *British Medical Journal*, **281**: 879-89.
21. Sivenius, J., Meraca, K., Heinonen, O.P. *et al.* (1985). The significance of intensive rehabilitation of stroke: A controlled trial. *Stroke*, **16**: 928-31.

Chapter 10: Technology assessment

1. Donabedian, G. (1988). The assessment of technology and quality: A comparative study of certainties and ambiguities. *International Journal of Technology Assessment in Health Care*, 4 (4): 487-96.
2. Schon, D.A. (1987). *Technology and Change*. De la corte Press, New York.
3. Stocking, B. (1985). *Initiative and Inertia*. The Nuffield Provincial Hospitals Trust, London.

4. Greer, A.L. (1987). Rationing medical technology. *International Journal of Technology Assessment in Health Care*, 3: 199–222.
5. Peddecord, K.M., Janon, E.A. and Robins, J.M. (1988). Substitution of magnetic resonance imaging for computed tomography. *International Journal of Technology Assessment in Health Care*, 4(4): 573–91.
6. Battista, R.N. (1989). Innovation and diffusion of health related technologies. *International Journal of Technology Assessment in Health Care*, 5(2): 227–48.
7. Harrison, S. (1988). *Managing the National Health Service, Shifting the Frontier?* Chapman and Hall, London.
8. Etzioni, A. (1964). *Modern Organizations*. Prentice-Hall, Englewood Cliffs, N.J.
9. Child, J. (1984). *Organisation*. Harper and Row, London.
10. Guest, R.H., Hersey, P. and Blanchard, K.H. (1986). *Organisational Change Through Effective Leadership*. Prentice-Hall, Englewood Cliffs, N.J.
11. Handy, C.B. (1985). *Understanding Organisations*. Penguin, Harmondsworth.
12. Donabedian, A. (1980). *Explorations in Quality Assessment and Monitoring: Vol. 1. The Definition of Quality and Approaches to Its Assessment*. Health Administration Press, Ann Arbor, Mich.
13. Challah, S. and Mays, N.B. (1986). The randomised controlled trial in the evaluation of new technology: A case study. *British Medical Journal*, 292: 877–9.
14. Tymstra, T. (1989). The imperative character of medical technology and the meaning of 'anticipated decision regret'. *International Journal of Technology Assessment in Health Care*, 5(2): 207–13.
15. Miller, E., Ashworth, L.A.E., Robinson, A. *et al.* (1991). Phase II trial of whole-cell pertussis vaccine vs an acellular vaccine containing agglutinogens. *Lancet*, 337: 70–73.
16. Bailey, F.G. (1990). *Strategies and Spoils: A Social Anthropology of Politics*. Blackwell, Oxford.
17. Cooper, L.S., Chalmers, T.C., McCally, M. *et al.* (1988). The poor quality of early evaluation of magnetic resonance imaging. *Journal of the American Medical Association*, 259: 3277–80.
18. Grant, J.M. (1991). The fetal heart rate trace is normal, isn't it? Observer agreement of categorical assessment. *Lancet*, 337: 215–18.
19. Klazinga, N. (1990). *Technology assessment and quality assurance applied sciences in health care management*. Paper presented at ISTA, 21 May 1990, Houston, Texas.
20. Elliot, S.J. (1991). Neonatal extracorporeal membrane oxygenation: How not to assess novel technologies. *Lancet*, 337: 476–8.

Chapter 11: Important methodological issues

1. Abramson, J.H. (1986). *Survey Methods in Community Medicine: An Introduction to Epidemiological and Evaluative Studies*, 3rd edn. Churchill Livingstone, London.
2. Siegel, S. and Castellan, N.J. (1989). *Non-parametric Statistics for the Behavioural Sciences*, 2nd edn. McGraw-Hill, New York.
3. Oldham, P.D. (1962). A note on the analysis of repeated measurements of the same subjects. *Journal of Chronic Disease*, 15: 969.
4. Press, W.H., Flannery, B.P., Teukolsky, S.A. *et al.* (1988). *Numerical Recipes in C: The Art of Scientific Computing*. Cambridge University Press, Cambridge. (There are also editions of this work for the FORTRAN and Pascal computer languages.)
5. Goodman, S.N. (1989). Meta-analysis and evidence. *Controlled Clinical Trials*, 10: 188–204.

6. Gotzsche, P.D. (1989). Meta-analysis of grip strength: Most common, but superfluous variable in comparative NSAID trials. *Danish Medical Bulletin*, 36: 393-5.
7. Libretti, A. and Bertele, V. (1989). Antiplatelet drugs in secondary prevention of myocardial infarction: Clinical recommendations and perspective implications. *Journal of Cardiovascular Pharmacology*, 14: S89-91 (suppl. 9).
8. Henderson, W.G., Goldman, S., Copeland, J.G. *et al.* (1989). Antiplatelet or anticoagulant therapy after coronary bypass surgery: A meta-analysis of clinical trials. *Annals of Internal Medicine*, 111: 743-50.

Chapter 12: Making evaluation work

1. March, J.G. (1984). Theories of choice and making decisions. In R. Paton (ed.), *Organisations: Cases, Issues, Concepts*. Harper and Row, London, pp. 91-7.
2. Schnieden, H. and Grimes, M. (1989). Audit and performance indicators: A case study in ophthalmology. *Journal of Management in Medicine*, 3: 301-14.
3. James, W. (1907). *Pragmatism: A New Name for Some Old Ways of Thinking*. Longmans, Green and Co., London.
4. Machiavelli, N. (1973). *The Prince* (translated by G. Ball). Penguin, Harmondsworth.
5. Roberts, J. (1991). Navigating the seas of change. *British Medical Journal*, 302: 34-7.
6. Department of Health and Social Security (1982). *Steering Group on Health Services Information 1st Report to the Secretary of State* (the Korner Report). HMSO, London.
7. Pickin, C. and St Leger, A.S. (1990). *Assessment of Health Need Using the Life Cycle Framework: An Information Toolbox*. North Western Regional Health Authority, Manchester.
8. St Leger, A.S., Allen, D. and Rowsell, K.V. (1989). Procedures for evaluating innovatory proposals. *British Medical Journal*, 299: 1017-18.
9. Patel, M.S., St Leger, A.S. and Schnieden, H. (1985). Process and outcome in the National Health Service. *British Medical Journal*, 291: 1365-6.

Further reading

Accreditation and quality assurance
Borus, M.E., Buntz, C.G. and Tash, W.R. (1982). *Evaluating the Impact of Health Programs: A Primer*. MIT Press, Cambridge, Mass.

Kings Fund (1990). *Organisational Audit (Accreditation UK)*. Kings Fund, London.

Wilson, C.R.M. (1987). *Hospital Wide Quality Assurance*. W.B. Saunders, distributed by Harcourt Brace Jovanonvich, London.

World Health Organization (1989). *Quality Assurance in Health Care*, Vol. 1, No. 2/3, WHO, Geneva.

Audit
Hopkins, A. and Costain, D. (1990). *Measuring the Outcomes of Medical Care*. Royal College of Physicians, London.

Shaw, C. (1989). *Medical Audit: A Hospital Handbook*. Kings Fund, London. (An excellent introduction to audit)

Clinical trials
Peto, R., Pike, M.C., Armitage, P. *et al.* (1976). Design and analysis of randomized clinical trials requiring prolonged observation of each patient: I. Introduction and design. *British Journal of Cancer*, 34: 585–612.

Peto, R., Pike, M.C., Armitage, P. *et al.* (1977). Design and analysis of randomized clinical trials requiring prolonged observation of each patient: II. Analysis and examples. *British Journal of Cancer*, 35: 1–39.

Pocock, S.J.P. (1983). *Clinical Trials: A Practical Approach*. John Wiley, Chichester. (Highly recommended)

Epidemiology
Last, J.M. (ed.) (1988). *A Dictionary of Epidemiology*. Oxford University Press, Oxford.

Evaluation, general
Cochrane, A.L. (1972) *Effectiveness and Efficiency: Random Reflections on Health Services*. Nuffield Provincial Hospitals Trust, London. (A classic work which every health professional should read)

Donabedian, A. (1980, 1982, 1985). *Explorations in Quality Assessment and Monitoring*. Vol. 1: *The Definition of Quality and Approaches to its Assessment*;

Vol. 2: *The Criteria and Standards of Quality*; Vol. 3: *The Methods and Findings of Quality Assessment and Monitoring: An Illustrated Analysis*. Health Administration Press, Ann Arbor, Mich. (These volumes comprise the major recent work in this field)
Holland, W.W. (ed.) (1983). *Evaluation of Health Care*. Oxford University Press, Oxford. (Contains interesting examples of evaluation studies)

Health economics
Ashmore, M., Mulkay, M. and Pinch, T. (1989). *Health and Efficiency: A Sociology of Health Economics*. Open University Press, Milton Keynes.
Calvo, P. and Wough, G. (1977). *Micro-economics: An Introductory Text*. McGraw-Hill, Sydney.
Culyer, A.J. (1985). *Health Service Efficiency: Appraising the Appraisers*. Discussion Paper No. 10, Centre for Health Economics, University of York.
Department of Health and Social Security (1986). *Breast Cancer Screening*. HMSO, London. (Pages 52 and 65 are a useful model of a good economic appraisal)
Drummond, M.F. (1990). Allocating resources. *International Journal of Technology Assessment in Health Care*, 6 (1): 77–92.
Drummond, M.F., Stoddard, G.L. and Torrance, G.W. (1987). *Methods for the Economic Evaluation of Health Care Programmes*. Oxford University Press, Oxford. (A particularly clear and useful work for the practitioner of evaluation)
Jones-Lee, M.W. (ed.) (1982). *The Value of Life and Safety*. North-Holland, Oxford.
Luce, B.R. and Elixhauser, A. (1990). Estimating costs in the economic evaluation of medical technologies. *International Journal of Technology Assessment in Health Care*, 6 (1): 57–76.
Torrance, G.W. and Feeny, D. (1989). Utilities and quality-adjusted life years. *International Journal of Technology Assessment in Health Care*, 5 (3): 559–75.

The NHS
Strong, P. and Robinson, J. (1990). *The NHS: Under New Management*. Open University Press, Milton Keynes.

Philosophy of science
Chalmers, A. (1990). *Science and its Fabrication*. Open University Press, Milton Keynes.
Feyerabend, P.F. (1984). *Against Method: Outline of an Anarchistic Theory of Knowledge*. Verso, London. (A classic but not easy)
Kuhn, T.S. (1970). *The Structure of Scientific Revolutions*, 2nd edn. University of Chicago Press, Chicago, Ill. (A classic but not easy)
Medawar, P.B. (1970). *Induction and Intuition in Scientific Thought*. Methuen, London. (A splendid introduction to those new to this field)
Popper, K.R. (1974). *The Logic of Scientific Discovery*. Hutchinson, London. (Inspirational but not easy)

Quality of life
Bowling, A. (1991). *Measuring Health: A Review of Quality of Life Measurement Scales*. Open University Press, Milton Keynes.
McDowell, I. and Newall, C. (1987). *Measuring Health: A Guide to Rating Scales and Questionnaires*. Oxford University Press, Oxford.
Walker, S.R. and Rosser, R.M. (eds) (1987). *Quality of Life Assessment and its Applications*. MTP Press, Dordrecht, Netherlands.

Statistics

Armitage, P. and Berry, G. (1987). *Statistical Methods in Medical Research*, 2nd edn. Blackwell, Oxford. (Excellent bench book for evaluators)

Gardner, M.J. and Altman, D.G. (eds) (1989). Statistics with confidence. *British Medical Journal*. (Very useful and written at an elementary level)

Kendall, M.G. and Buckland, W.R. (1983). *Dictionary of Statistical Terms*. Longman, London.

Oldham, P.D. (1968). *Measurement in Medicine: The Interpretation of Numerical Data*. The English Universities Press, London. (A classic)

Woodward, M. and Francis, L.M. (1988). *Statistics for Health Management and Research*. Edward Arnold, London. (Recommended)

Survey methods

Abramson, J.H. (1986). *Survey Methods in Community Medicine: An Introduction to Epidemiological and Evaluative Studies*, 3rd edn. Churchill Livingstone, London. (Excellent and easily accessible to those who have understood our Chapter 11)

Moser, C.A. and Kacton, G. (1986). *Survey Methods in Social Investigation*. Gower, London.

Sutton, C. (1987). *A Handbook of Research for the Helping Professions*. Routledge and Kegan Paul, London.